Ulcerative Colitis and Crohn's Disease
A Clinician's Guide

Ulcerative Colitis and Crohn's Disease
A Clinician's Guide

By

D. P. Jewell MA DPhil FRCP

Consultant Physician, John Radcliffe Hospital, Oxford; Clinical Lecturer, Oxford University, Oxford, UK

R. W. G. Chapman MD MRCP

Consultant Physician, John Radcliffe Hospital, Oxford, UK

N. Mortensen MD FRCS

Consultant Surgeon, John Radcliffe Hospital, Oxford, UK

CHURCHILL LIVINGSTONE
EDINBURGH LONDON MADRID MELBOURNE NEW YORK AND TOKYO 1992

CHURCHILL LIVINGSTONE
Medical Division of Longman Group UK Limited

Distributed in the United States of America by Churchill
Livingstone Inc., 650 Avenue of the Americas, New York,
N.Y. 10011, and by associated companies, branches and
representatives throughout the world.

First published 1992

ISBN 0-443-04803-7

British Library Cataloguing in Publication Data
A catalogue record for this book is available from the British
Library

Library of Congress Cataloging in Publication Data is
available

Printed in Great Britain by George Over Limited,
London and Rugby

Preface

Ulcerative colitis and Crohn's disease represent two of the major challenges in gastroenterology today. Their pathogenesis is poorly understood, we do not know their aetiology, and we are unable to describe their genetic implications with any precision. From the patient's point-of-view, both diseases may give rise to considerable morbidity, the side-effects of medical treatment are often unpleasant, and surgery is frequently necessary.

In this book we have tried to provide a clinical account of the two diseases and their management for physicians and surgeons who have to look after patients with these disorders, but who are not specialists in this field. The aim has been to concentrate on how these diseases present and how they are managed, both medically and surgically. It was not intended to provide a detailed review — many of these already exist and at the end of each chapter some key references are provided which should allow the reader ready access to the literature. One of the more important developments in recent years has been the establishment of patient self-help groups. These have provided considerable support for patients and have had a major impact on education and understanding. For many patients, membership of one of these groups is an important contribution to their overall management. Thus, the addresses of these organizations, as well as other charitable organizations specifically interested in this area, are provided at the end of the book.

In preparing the manuscript, we acknowledge the very great help provided by Dr D J Nolan and Dr A Campbell in respectively selecting the radiological and histopathological illustrations. We are also very grateful to our secretaries, Mrs E Clarke and Miss C Cullen, for the hours of over-time it has taken to prepare the text for publication.

Oxford
1992

D.P.J.
R.W.G.C.
N.M.

Contents

1. Definition and history   1

2. Epidemiology   6

3. Aetiology and pathogenesis   9

4. Clinical features   14

5. Investigations and differential diagnosis   21

6. Extraintestinal manifestations of inflammatory bowel disease   42

7. Medical management   49

8. Surgical treatment   58

9. Prognosis   69

Useful addresses   75

Index   76

1 Definition and history

DEFINITION

Inflammatory bowel disease is, by common usage, a collective term describing ulcerative colitis and Crohn's disease. It is a term that is imprecise and therefore best avoided because many other inflammatory conditions are known to affect both the small and large intestine.

Ulcerative colitis is a diffuse inflammatory disorder of the colon which always affects the rectum and extends proximally, in continuity, to involve a variable degree of the rest of the bowel (Fig. 1.1). The disease process always stops in the caecum and does not involve the small intestine. Histologically, there is an acute inflammatory infiltrate in the colonic lamina propria consisting of neutrophils, eosinophils and plasma cells and, characteristically, the neutrophils

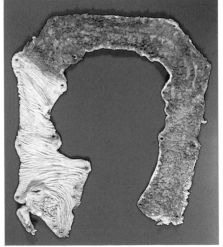

Fig. 1.1 A colon resected for severe ulcerative colitis. There is sparing of the right colon but the remainder is severely inflamed with longitudinal ulceration.

1

are seen penetrating the epithelial cells of the crypts with the formation of crypt abscesses (Fig. 1.2). The changes of more chronic disease are usually seen, such as disturbance of gland architecture and a lymphocytic infiltrate.

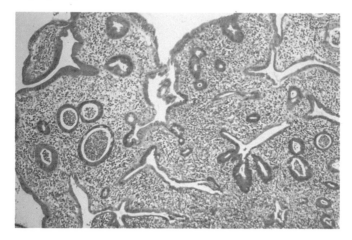

Fig. 1.2   Histological appearances of active ulcerative colitis. There is pseudo-polypoid change, a dense inflammatory infiltrate, loss of goblet cells and crypt abscess formation.

In contrast, Crohn's disease can affect any part of the gastrointestinal tract. Most commonly, it is seen in the ileocaecal region (Fig. 1.3) but it can be confined to the anus or, rarely, to the mouth. It is a

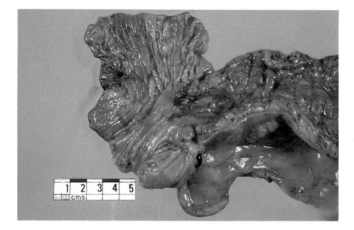

Fig. 1.3   Ileocaecal resection specimen from a patient with Crohn's disease. The terminal ileum shows thickening of the wall, and an oedematous, ulcerated mucosa.

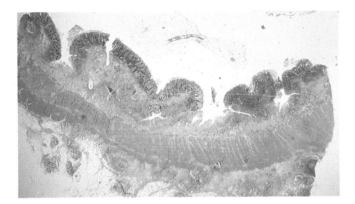

Fig. 1.4 Microscopic appearances of Crohn's disease of the colon showing fissure ulcers and a transmural inflammation extending to the serosa which contains granulomas.

disease that may involve several segments of the intestine simultaneously ('skip lesions'), the intervening bowel being histologically normal, and it is frequently associated either with stricturing or with fistula formation into adjacent loops of intestine or into the bladder or vagina. Histologically, the inflammatory infiltrate is transmucosal and consists predominantly of lymphocytes, plasma cells and macrophages (Fig. 1.4). The hallmark of Crohn's disease is the granuloma (Fig. 1.5), which often contains giant cells; however, it

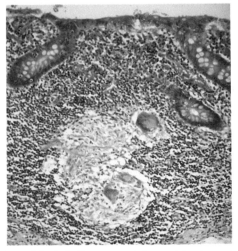

Fig. 1.5 Granuloma of Crohn's disease containing multinucleate giant cells. The surrounding mucosa is heavily infiltrated with lymphocytes and plasma cells.

is present in only 3–4% of cases. There is accumulating evidence, based on quantitative histological morphometry and enzyme studies, that the whole of the intestinal tract may be abnormal in patients with Crohn's disease.

Both ulcerative colitis and Crohn's disease are chronic disorders; most patients suffer intermittent relapses of their disease.

HISTORY

In 1859, Samuel Wilks, a physician at Guy's Hospital in London, described 'The morbid appearances of the colon of Miss Bankes' following an autopsy performed on a patient who had died with a blood diarrhoea. He recognized that this condition was different from a dysenteric illness (greatly prevalent at the time) and, in the same year, he reported on a series of patients with similar clinical features for which he used the term 'ulcerative colitis'. There was considerable debate over whether this was a distinct entity or a manifestation of dysentery but, by the 1920s, Sir Arthur Hurst was able to describe all major clinical features of the disease as we know it today.

Crohn's disease derives its name from the description of eight cases of regional ileitis described by Crohn, Ginsburg and Oppenheimer in 1932. However, the first clear description of the disease and the recognition that the granulomatous inflammation was not due to tuberculosis was made by Dalziel in 1912. The earlier term of regional ileitis was replaced by regional enteritis in 1951 when it was recognized by Lockhart-Mummery and Morson that the disease was not confined to the ileum when they described primary Crohn's disease of the colon. This entity was subsequently termed granulomatous colitis by American clinicians. With such a profusion of names, it is probably preferable to use 'Crohn's disease' to describe all forms of the disease.

Clinical, radiological and histological criteria have now been determined to distinguish ulcerative colitis and Crohn's disease. Nevertheless, in a few patients, diagnostic doubt may remain and these cases are described as 'colitis indeterminate'.

The introduction of corticosteroids in the late 1940s and early 1950s has had a major impact on the outlook of severe attacks of both diseases. Combined with better management of fluid and electrolyte balance and improvements in surgical technique, this has led to a reduction of mortality from 45% in the pre-steroid era to less than

2% for patients suffering severe attacks of ulcerative colitis seen at specialist centres (this figure includes the operative mortality).

Management is unlikely to be completely successful until the aetiology and pathogenesis of the inflammatory process are understood. Until such time, it is not possible to be certain whether these two diseases are distinct entities or whether they represent the spectrum of a common pathology. At present, it is preferable to discuss the epidemiology, clinical features and management separately, as if the diseases were different.

2 Epidemiology

Although ulcerative colitis and Crohn's disease are both rare diseases, there appears to have been a gradual increase in incidence since the Second World War, especially in Crohn's disease. Despite improvements in the accuracy of diagnosis and of reporting, this increase does seem to be genuine.

INCIDENCE AND PREVALENCE

For ulcerative colitis, the incidence in northern Europe and the USA is between five and eight new cases per 100000 population per year, although figures tend to vary according to whether patients with proctitis are included. The prevalence of the disease is 80–90 per 100000 population. Prevalence is probably similar for Australasians and white South Africans, but the disease seems to be less common in eastern and southern Europe. So far, no reliable epidemiological studies covering Asia or South America have been published; however, the disease is now recognized in these areas and distinguished from bacillary dysentery. Data from Japan suggest that the disease is about ten times less common than it is in Europe or the USA. It is not clear whether the incidence of ulcerative colitis is increasing. In Scandinavia and Minnesota, USA, the incidence has roughly doubled in the last 50 years but at least some of this rise might be attributable to better diagnosis.

Crohn's disease is less common than ulcerative colitis. For northern Europe, the incidence is 2.0–4.5 per 100000 per year with a prevalence of 35–45 per 100000 population. In eastern and southern Europe and Japan, there is a low incidence of this disease. It appears to be extremely rare in Asia and South America, but diagnosis can be exceptionally difficult in countries where intestinal tuberculosis is common. The rise in the incidence of Crohn's disease over the last

40–50 years has been well documented in the UK and Sweden; there is a suggestion, which is not yet firmly established, that the rise may have reached a plateau and the incidence may now be declining.

To place these figures in perspective, a general practitioner in the UK with a list of 2500 patients can expect to look after two patients with ulcerative colitis and one with Crohn's disease.

Age and sex

Ulcerative colitis is slightly more common in women than in men, but the difference is small. For Crohn's disease, the sex ratio is about equal although there is considerable variability from one series to another. The peak age of onset for both diseases is in young adult life (20–40 years). However, virtually any age group can be affected and either disease may present, albeit rarely, within the first year of life or in the eighth decade. It has been suggested that there is a secondary peak of onset in the elderly, but this is as yet unproven.

Social class

Although a weak association between Crohn's disease and higher educational attainment has been reported, most studies have shown no difference in incidence among the social classes. However, there are known differences in smoking habit and the use of oral contraceptives among the social classes which may have a bearing on the pathogenesis of each disease (see Ch. 3).

Ethnic associations

The incidence of both diseases is higher in Jews in the USA and northern Europe than in those living in Israel. However, the incidence within Israel is variable: the highest rates are seen in Ashkenazi Jews who were born in the USA or Europe; low incidence rates are found in Israeli-born or non-Ashkenazi Jews. These findings strongly suggest that environmental factors are important in pathogenesis.

Although Crohn's disease seems to be rare in India, Asians emigrating to Europe or the USA appear susceptible to the disease. North American blacks also have a lower incidence of ulcerative colitis and of Crohn's disease; it is probably about 20–30% less than that of the white population.

CONCLUSIONS

Ulcerative colitis and Crohn's disease occur throughout the world but there are wide geographical variations in incidence, especially for Crohn's disease. The increasing incidence of Crohn's disease, together with the susceptibility of Asians living in the West and of the Western-born Jews, strongly suggests that environmental factors may be influencing the disease. However, the absence of clustering of cases, in space or time, makes a direct infective aetiology unlikely.

FURTHER READING

Mendeloff A I, Calkins B M 1988 The epidemiology of idiopathic inflammatory bowel disease. In: Kirsner J B, Shorter R G (eds) Inflammatory bowel disease, 3rd ed. Lea and Febiger, Philadelphia, pp 3–34

3 Aetiology and pathogenesis

The aetiology of either ulcerative colitis or Crohn's disease is not known but, even if ultimately a single initiating factor is found for each disease, the expression of the disease is likely to be multifactorial depending on the interplay of genetic and environmental factors. It is not clear whether the initiating factors are external (e.g., an infective agent) or whether the diseases represent a breakdown in mucosal defence mechanisms. However, there is some evidence to support the concept that the basic abnormality lies within the metabolism of the epithelial cell. Finally, continuous activation of the mucosal immune system may play a role in establishing the chronic nature of the diseases.

GENETIC FACTORS

The familial incidence of both Crohn's disease and ulcerative colitis is 10–15%, occurring predominantly in first-degree relatives. Both diseases can be represented in a single family but there is no single Mendelian pattern of inheritance. Furthermore, there is no close association with any of the HLA antigens except in Japan, where patients with ulcerative colitis are weakly linked with HLA-DR2. The results of studies in twin pairs suggest a stronger genetic element for Crohn's disease than for ulcerative colitis.

ENVIRONMENTAL FACTORS

Infective agents

For ulcerative colitis, there is no evidence for an infective agent, either bacterial or viral. For Crohn's disease, interest has been focused on many organisms, including RNA viruses and cell wall-deficient organisms. Current interest centres around an atypical mycobacterium. After many months of culture, such an organism has been grown from homogenates of Crohn's tissue and, when fed to neonatal goats, it caused an intestinal granulomatous inflammation. However, it has been isolated from only a minority of patients and disease specificity has not yet been adequately proven. Nevertheless, the techniques of molecular biology have shown that the organisms that have been isolated are identical to *Mycobacterium paratuberculosis*. This is the organism that causes Johne's disease in farm animals, which is a granulomatous disorder of the intestine. Thus, *M. paratuberculosis* might well be a candidate organism for Crohn's disease but the case is far from proven on current evidence.

Diet

Milk-free diets for patients with ulcerative colitis may reduce the relapse rate of the disease but the effect is marginal. In patients with Crohn's disease, there is more evidence that dietary factors may play a role. Although those patients with Crohn's disease, but not those with ulcerative colitis, have been shown to consume more sugar and less fibre than healthy subjects, a controlled trial of a low-sugar, high-fibre diet failed to show any benefit of this diet over a two-year period. However, active Crohn's disease may heal if the patient is treated with an elemental diet (glucose, amino acids), which is apparently as effective as treatment with corticosteroids. Thus, changing the nature of luminal contents may influence the disease, but whether this is brought about by reducing the antigenic load, by altering the luminal flora or by some other mechanism is not known.

Smoking habit

The findings of many studies have shown that non-smokers have a two- to sixfold increase in the incidence of ulcerative colitis when compared with smokers. In contrast, Crohn's disease occurs more commonly in smokers, with a relative risk of two to four. These findings are consistent among different centres, but the mechanisms involved are obscure. It is possible that, given a susceptibility towards developing intestinal inflammation, smoking habits may partly influence the nature of that inflammation.

Oral contraceptive pill

The results of prospective studies have shown that women on the oral contraceptive pill are more likely to develop ulcerative colitis or Crohn's disease than women using other forms of contraception.

The relative risk is small (1.5–2.0) and the statistical significance of the association is lost when corrections are made for smoking habit and social class.

Impaired epithelial cell function

Patients with either disease have been reported to have increased intestinal permeability even when in complete remission. For those with Crohn's disease, it may be seen in their first-degree relatives, although this is controversial as the initial observation has not been confirmed. This suggests that there may be an abnormality within the epithelial cell layer, a hypothesis that receives further support from the demonstration of an abnormal glycoprotein composition of the colonic mucus in patients who have ulcerative colitis. In metabolic studies using isolated colonic epithelial cells from patients with ulcerative colitis, an impaired facility to metabolize short-chain fatty acids, which form the major fuel for these cells, was found. Therefore, it is possible that, in ulcerative colitis at least, the colonic epithelial cells are abnormal, thereby leading to a deficient mucus layer and hence increased mucosal permeability. The nature of this defect could be under genetic control. Unfortunately, even in remission, the epithelial cells have a shorter half-life than normal so it is possible that these abnormalities of function may merely reflect a younger population of cells.

Immunological findings

Patients with both diseases show humoral and cellular immune responses to a variety of gut-associated antigens, including dietary proteins, and bacterial and epithelial cell antigens.

Furthermore, both peripheral blood and mucosal lymphocytes are cytotoxic to colonic epithelial cells in vitro, a phenomenon not displayed by lymphocytes from healthy subjects or from patients with diverticulitis. The question is whether these responses are merely secondary phenomena or whether they are pathogenetic.

The inflamed mucosa shows a striking increase in plasma cells producing immunoglobulin G (IgG) or IgM, some of which has antibody specificity for bacterial and possibly epithelial antigens. There is indirect evidence for complement activation; therefore it seems likely that antigen–antibody reactions with the activation of complement are a major mechanism for the inflammation. An attractive hypothesis for the establishment of chronic disease is that there is continuing stimulation of the local immune response leading to chronic activation of immune effector mechanisms, such as complement or T-cell cytotoxicity. Indeed, the many immunological responses to the gut-associated antigens may be a reflection of this process. Several mechanisms for such hyper-responsiveness have been suggested and include the following.

Antigen presentation by the epithelial cell

For T-helper cells to recognize an antigen, that antigen has to be 'processed' by an antigen-presenting cell displaying HLA-DR molecules on its surface, because the T-cell will 'see' the antigen only in the context of these HLA molecules. Normal colonic epithelium does not express HLA-DR molecules but expression does occur in the presence of inflammation. Thus, the epithelial cells might then be able to behave as antigen-presenting cells, which might lead to a marked increase in mucosal immune activation. However, as HLA-DR expression occurs in infective colitis, which is often self-limiting, this suggested mechanism cannot be the complete answer.

Disturbance of immunoregulatory control

This could occur because of a defect in T-suppressor cell activity which would allow an uncontrolled interaction between T-helper cells and B-cells, resulting in increased antibody synthesis. Unfortunately, the results of studies investigating suppressor or helper cell function have been highly variable and it seems unlikely that there is a major defect in immunoregulatory control. However, in a recent report, it was suggested that normal epithelial cells are able to activate suppressor T-cells within the epithelium (T-suppressor cells form 90–95% of the intra-epithelial lymphocytes) but that this mechanism does not occur in ulcerative colitis. Hence, not only would the inflamed epithelial cell (expressing HLA-DR molecules) present antigen to the underlying T-helper cells, but this process would proceed without the modulating influence of the intraepithelial suppressor cells.

Consequences of immune activation

Although the exact mechanisms may be unknown, there is little doubt that both humoral and cellular immune pathways are activated in the inflamed mucosa. This results in the release of a wide variety of cytokines from macrophages and T-cells, which serves not only to amplify the immune response but will induce an acute-phase response and will also lead to tissue injury, initiation of repair mechanisms and stimulation of fibrosis. Furthermore, many inflammatory mediators will be released from activated macrophages, eosinophils, mast cells and neutrophils, including leukotrienes, platelet-activating factor, reactive oxygen metabolites, kinins and other vasoactive substances. Together with the cytokines, these mediators will lead to increased epithelial and endothelial permeability, recruitment of inflammatory cells (which will themselves become activated), local ischaemia and tissue damage.

FURTHER READING

Boughton-Smith N, Pettipher R 1990 Lipid mediators and cytokines in inflammatory bowel disease. Eur J Gastroenterol Hepatol 2: 241–245

Lowes J R, Jewell D P 1990 Immunology of inflammatory bowel disease. Semin Immunopathol 12: 251–268

McConnell R B 1990 Genetics of inflammatory bowel disease. In: Allan R N, Keighley M R B, Alexander-Williams J, Hawkins C F (eds) Inflammatory bowel diseases, 2nd edn. Churchill Livingstone, Edinburgh pp 11–23

4 Clinical features

Although the clinical features of ulcerative colitis and Crohn's disease can be very similar, they are often sufficiently distinctive to allow the differential diagnosis to be made. Therefore, each disease will be considered separately.

ULCERATIVE COLITIS

Ulcerative colitis always begins in the rectum and extends proximally to involve a variable length of the colon, but it never extends beyond the ileocaecal valve. In approximately 30% of patients, only the rectum or rectosigmoid will be involved, 20% will have total colitis and the rest (50%) will have varying degrees of involvement of the colon. It is not uncommon to find that patients can be completely asymptomatic even though endoscopic examination shows diffuse inflammation.

Symptoms

The major symptoms are rectal bleeding, diarrhoea, the passage of mucus and abdominal pain, mentioned in order of frequency of occurrence. Usually, symptoms develop gradually but occasionally they can seem to start abruptly, often simulating an infection.

Patients with inflammation confined to the rectum (haemorrhagic proctitis) may present with constipation with fresh blood on the stool, a clinical picture similar to that of haemorrhoids.

However, if more extensive inflammation is present, patients complain of severe disabling diarrhoea. Nocturnal diarrhoea is common and the symptoms of urgency and tenesmus are usually present. Blood and mucus are usually mixed with the stool. If a fulminant colitis is present, the blood is mixed with pus and liquid stool, and appears brownish, rather like anchovy sauce. Patients often do not recognize this as blood and may deny passing blood, which can mislead the doctor taking the history. Pain is not a prominent symptom for most patients who have ulcerative colitis, but mild colic and lower abdominal discomfort relieved by defaecation are present in some. More severe pain can occur during severe attacks.

Other symptoms include lethargy and general malaise and symptoms of anaemia, such as tiredness, swollen ankles and shortness of breath. Weight loss is common in more severe disease and is partly due to anorexia and nausea, which may be accompanying symptoms, and partly due to protein loss and hypercatabolism. Patients may also complain of symptoms related to the extraintestinal manifestations of ulcerative colitis (see Ch. 6).

Physical signs

Patients who have distal disease, especially if it is only mildly active, appear to be well and there are no abnormal physical signs. If the disease is more active, the descending colon may be tender on palpation.

Patients with more severe disease can also look surprisingly well, having few signs, which often misleads the inexperienced doctor into underestimating the disease activity. However, in a fulminating attack, the patient usually looks ill with evidence of weight loss and salt and water depletion. Tachycardia is invariably present, and there may be a low blood pressure with a postural drop. Patients may be febrile and clinically anaemic, with signs of iron deficiency. Chronic disease is sometimes associated with finger clubbing, and patients with hypoproteinaemia may have oedema. Oral candidiasis can occur in severely ill patients.

With severe disease, abdominal examination reveals generalized tenderness along the length of the colon, often with rebound. The abdomen may be distended and tympanitic but it is usually flat. Bowel sounds can be reduced. Perianal disease is predominantly a feature of Crohn's disease although small fissures can occur in patients who have ulcerative colitis.

Assessment of severity

The clinical guide to severity was devised by Truelove and Witts for the initial cortisone trial and it remains clinically useful. The criteria are as follows:

Mild: less than four motions daily, usually with blood. No evidence of systemic disturbance.

Moderate: less than eight motions daily, with blood. No systemic disturbance.

Severe: eight or more stools daily with evidence of systemic illness as shown by fever, anaemia, tachycardia, high erythrocyte sedimentation rate, hypokalaemia.

Complications

There may be systemic and local complications associated with a severe attack of ulcerative colitis. The systemic complications include water and electrolyte imbalance, septicaemia and thromboembolism. The local complications are an acute dilatation of the colon, perforation and massive haemorrhage.

Water and electrolyte deficiencies

The severe diarrhoea leads to losses of sodium, potassium and water. If the attack is promptly and effectively treated (Ch. 7), these losses rarely cause clinical problems. Hypokalaemia is common and may be a trigger for an acute dilatation.

Septicaemia

Patients coming to surgery for severe attacks have been shown to have a high incidence of portal pyaemia. Nevertheless, a systemic septicaemia is uncommon. Blood cultures should always be taken but prophylactic antibiotics are not indicated unless perforation has occurred.

Thromboembolism

Thromboembolism is a dangerous complication associated with severe disease (see Ch. 6). If venous thrombosis occurs, it is usually safe to treat patients with anticoagulants using standard therapeutic regimes.

Acute dilatation

Acute dilatation occurs in about 10% of severe attacks. Although the mechanisms underlying the dilatation are not known, hypokalaemia and the administration of opiates may be precipitating factors. The earliest clinical sign of a dilating colon is usually a rise in pulse rate, abdominal girth increases and there is a reduction in bowel sounds.

Perforation

Perforation of a severely inflamed colon is uncommon. It is often associated with an acute dilatation but can occur in patients who do not have a dilated colon. Diagnosis may be delayed because the classical signs of colonic perforation and of faecal peritonitis may be absent, especially if the patient is receiving corticosteroid therapy. This complication should always be suspected if the pulse rises and the patient's condition worsens. Plain abdominal radiographs may show free air in the peritoneal cavity but absence of this sign does not exclude the diagnosis.

CROHN'S DISEASE

The clinical features of Crohn's disease are partly determined by the site of the disease. The majority of patients (45%) will have ileocaecal disease, but 30% will have only ileal disease and in 25% the disease is confined to the colon. Very rarely, a patient will present with Crohn's disease restricted to the mouth, oesophagus, stomach or anus. However, as few clinicians will ever see these patients, they will not be discussed further.

Symptoms

Symptoms are highly variable. Diarrhoea occurs in 70–90% of patients but rectal bleeding occurs in only about one-third. Abdominal pain is present in at least half of the patients, and the systemic symptoms of malaise, anorexia, fever and weight loss are common. Nausea and vomiting are frequently associated with severe disease. The clinical picture tends to differ according to the site of disease (Table 4.1). Thus, rectal bleeding usually signifies colonic disease, as do symptoms related to the extraintestinal manifestations (see Ch. 6). Colicky abdominal pain is more frequent with small intestinal disease, whereas the pain associated with colonic Crohn's disease is often more of a dull ache.

Table 4.1   Clinical presentation of Crohn's disease in relation to the predominant site of disease

Presentation	Site of disease (%)	
	Ileal	Colonic
Rectal bleeding	22	46
Abdominal pain	62	55
Malnutrition	19	22
Abdominal mass	8–30	0
Extraintestinal manifestations	1	20

Symptoms of pain, diarrhoea, vomiting and weight loss may indicate active disease but they may also indicate intestinal obstruction from stricture formation in the absence of active inflammation. Thus, the clinical assessment of these patients is not always straightforward.

Small intestinal disease may be associated with malabsorption, which is usually caused by bacterial overgrowth secondary to stasis. The diarrhoea may then have the features of steatorrhoea. Symptoms of anaemia are common but are usually due to iron deficiency from blood loss rather than malabsorption of the haematinics. Serum B_{12} concentrations can be low in patients with ileal disease but the neurological complications, such as subacute combined degeneration of the cord, are not seen. Symptoms of osteomalacia or vitamin K deficiency from malabsorption of the fat-soluble vitamins are also extremely uncommon.

In children, failure to thrive and stunting of growth are common presentations. In adults, presentation can occasionally be of fever and weight loss without gastrointestinal symptoms. Some patients, usually those with colonic disease, can present with the perianal complications of fistulae, fissures and abscesses.

Physical signs

Many patients will show evidence of weight loss or frank cachexia. They may be anaemic, with signs of iron deficiency, and show finger clubbing and the characteristic skin changes and oedema of hypoproteinaemia. Aphthous ulceration of the mouth is common. With severe disease, a tachycardia with a small-volume pulse, hypotension and fever are usually present. Abdominal examination may reveal thickened tender ileal loops in the right iliac fossa or there may be a frank inflammatory mass. Examination of the perineum and anus reveals lesions in at least 30% of patients. Fleshy violaceous skin tags are probably the commonest feature, but fissures and small fistulae opening out onto the buttocks adjacent to the anus are also common (Fig. 4.1). The opening of the fistulae are also fleshy and violaceous in colour and may be draining pus (Fig. 4.2). Rarely, there is ulceration and fistulation which can involve the whole perineum and can spread to involve the vulva or the scrotum.

Presentation

The majority of patients present with the symptoms and signs described above and the diagnosis is usually strongly suspected before the results of investigation are known.

About 10% of patients with Crohn's disease have been reported to present as an acute appendicitis but, at operation, are found to have an acute ileitis. However, long term follow-up studies have shown that the majority of these patients do not relapse and it seems unlikely that Crohn's disease was the cause of the acute ileitis – yersiniosis of a viral aetiology is more likely. Nevertheless, a few patients presenting in this way do have Crohn's disease and a careful history may reveal intermittent symptoms in the months preceding the acute episode.

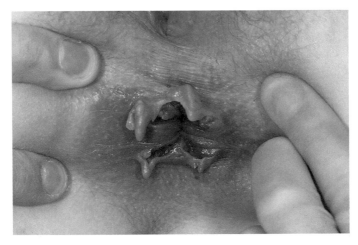

Fig. 4.1   Anal Crohn's disease showing multiple fissures.

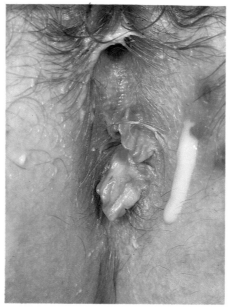

Fig. 4.2   Perianal fistulae in a patient with Crohn's disease.

The symptoms of variable bowel habit and abdominal pain in an otherwise well patient can be attributed to an irritable bowel syndrome, especially when the laboratory indicators of inflammation (erythrocyte sedimentation rate, C-reactive protein, platelets) are all normal. For these reasons, the mean time between presentation to a doctor and the diagnosis of Crohn's disease being made can be as long as three years. Hence, if there are any suspicious symptoms such as night-time diarrhoea or weight loss, the patient should be carefully investigated for Crohn's disease (Ch. 5).

FURTHER READING

Allan R N, Keighley M R B, Alexander-Williams J, Hawkins C F (eds) 1990 Inflammatory bowel diseases, 2nd edn. Churchill Livingstone, Edinburgh

Both H, Torp-Pedersen K, Kriener S, Hendriksen C, Binder V 1983 Clinical manifestations of ulcerative colitis and Crohn's disease in a regional patient group. Scand J Gastroenterol 18: 987–991

Kirsner J B, Shorter R G (eds) 1988 Inflammatory bowel disease, 3rd edn. Lea and Febiger, Philadelphia

Rao S C C, Holdsworth C D, Read N W 1988 Symptoms and stool patterns in patients with ulcerative colitis. Gut 29: 342–345

5 Investigations and differential diagnosis

The diagnosis of ulcerative colitis and of Crohn's disease is based on the clinical picture, combined with examination of the stool, laboratory investigations, endoscopic and radiological appearances and the histological assessment of rectal and colonic biopsies. The sequence of events in the investigation of patients with bloody diarrhoea is shown in Figure 5.1.

INVESTIGATION OF ULCERATIVE COLITIS

Stool examination

The macroscopic appearance of the stool in ulcerative colitis is very variable. Patients with inflammation confined to the rectum (proctitis) frequently pass hard, formed stools together with fresh blood and mucus. In contrast, patients with more widespread colonic inflammation produce liquid and semi-formed stools with blood and mucus. Microscopic examination of the stool in patients with active inflammation reveals large numbers of pus cells, and eosinophils are frequently seen. Stools should be cultured to exclude enteric pathogens including *Campylobacter jejuni* and *Clostridium difficile*. The presence of *Clostridium difficile* toxin must also be excluded. If there is any history of foreign travel, raising the suspicion of amoebiasis, fresh stools should be examined under the microscope within minutes of obtaining the specimen.

Laboratory investigations

Haematological and biochemical investigations are often normal in patients with mild or moderate attacks of acute ulcerative colitis. Patients with more severe attacks may become iron deficient; a hypochromic microcytic anaemia is often seen in these patients.

History	NB:	Antibiotics, foreign travel, systemic weight loss
General examination	NB:	Mouth ulcers, uveitis, arthropathy, erythema nodosum/pyoderma gangrenosum
Rectal examination	NB:	Skin tags, fistulae, fissures = Crohn's disease
Test stool for presence of blood		
Send stool to laboratory for microscopy and culture		
Rigid sigmoidoscopy	NB:	Charcoal swabs into Smart's medium if gonococcal infection suspected
Rectal biopsy (below 10 cm/posterior wall)		

Laboratory investigations

- Hb, WBC, ESR
- CRP/orosomucoid
- Liver function tests
- Renal function/ electrolytes

Consider

- Fe/TIBC; B_{12}, folate
- Infective serology: amoebae, *Yersinia*, *Chlamydia*
- HIV

Radiological investigations

Mild/moderate colitis   Severe colitis

- Barium enema   - Plain abdominal film

Consider

- Colonoscopy

Fig. 5.1   Flow diagram for the investigation of a patient with bloody diarrhoea.

Active inflammation is often associated with an elevated erythrocyte sedimentation rate (ESR), raised C-reactive protein and serum orosomucoid concentrations, and a thrombocytosis.

The serum albumin concentration is often low in severe attacks and can be used as a marker of disease severity. Transitory elevations of serum alkaline phosphatase and transaminases often occur in severe attacks, but these levels return to normal when the disease goes into remission. Approximately 3–5% of patients will have persistently abnormal liver function tests, usually an increased serum alkaline phosphatase. Such changes often indicate the presence of chronic hepatobiliary disease such as primary sclerosing cholangitis (Ch. 6).

Sigmoidoscopy

Sigmoidoscopy is essential in patients who have a diarrhoeal illness with rectal bleeding. This examination is best done without any bowel preparation because the early changes of acute ulcerative colitis can be mimicked by preparation enemas or washouts. The early sigmoidoscopic change of ulcerative colitis is loss of the mucosal vascular pattern, which appears reddened and oedematous, and thickening of the valves of Houston. The mucosa may have a granular appearance. More marked inflammation produces friability, so that gently touching the mucosa with a swab produces haemorrhage — 'contact bleeding'. In severe colitis, the mucosa may be bleeding spontaneously and there may be frank ulceration (Figs 5.2 and 5.3). Profuse amounts of bloody liquid stool may pour down from above, making sigmoidoscopy difficult for the inexperienced operator. In remission, the sigmoidoscopic appearances may return to normal, although in some patients with long-standing disease the mucosa may become atrophic in appearance.

Sigmoidoscopy will be abnormal in all patients who have active ulcerative colitis. Appearances can be misleading, however, in some patients who have been using topical therapy. In this group, the rectum can appear 'spared' although there may be severe proximal inflammation.

Radiology

In all patients suspected of having a severe attack of ulcerative colitis, erect and supine films of the abdomen should be taken. The films often reveal the extent of inflammation, showing thickening

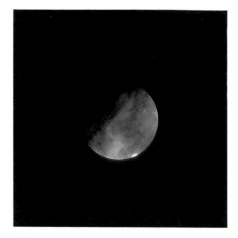

Fig. 5.2 Endoscopic appearances of moderately active ulcerative colitis showing an inflamed, friable mucosa.

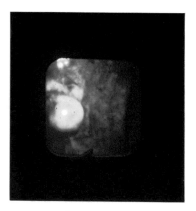

Fig. 5.3 Endoscopic appearances of severe ulcerative colitis with spontaneous bleeding. Note the inflammatory polyp.

and oedema of the bowel wall. Moreover, the extent of inflammation can often be judged from the presence of faeces in the proximal colon, as the inflamed segment of colon does not contain faecal matter (Fig. 5.4). In patients with a total colitis, there may be no

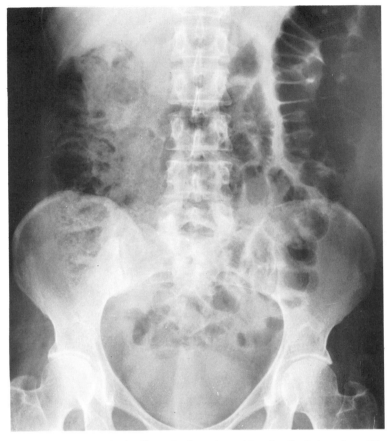

Fig. 5.4   Plain abdominal radiograph of a patient with active distal ulcerative colitis showing proximal constipation.

faeces visible on the radiograph. In more severe cases, the normal colonic haustral pattern is lost and the colon dilates (Fig. 5.5). Acute toxic dilatation should be suspected if the colonic diameter becomes greater than 5.5 cm. In the severest cases, mucosal islands (Fig. 5.5) can be seen on the plain abdominal X-ray. This sign represents islands of epithelium surrounded by an ulcerated mucosa and indicates that the patient is very likely to fail medical treatment and will require urgent colectomy. The plain abdominal X-ray will also exclude a colonic perforation. Double-contrast barium enemas must be avoided in patients who have severe colitis because of the risk of perforation. If the diagnosis is in doubt, an instant barium enema

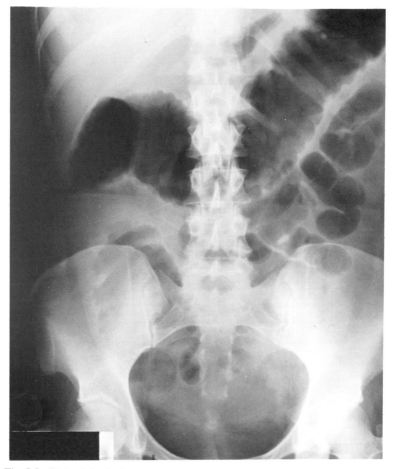

Fig. 5.5 Plain abdominal radiograph of a patient with severe ulcerative colitis affecting the whole colon. The transverse colon is dilated and shows mucosal islands indicating severe ulceration.

can be performed. In this procedure, barium is run carefully into the unprepared colon, without insufflation of air. This technique is rarely indicated and should only be carried out by an experienced radiologist.

In patients with mild or moderately active disease, a double-contrast barium enema can be performed safely. The radiographic appearances of the mucosa vary from a granular appearance with a thickened indistinct mucosal line, to deep ulceration (Figs 5.6 and 5.7). In patients with long-standing disease, the haustral pattern is

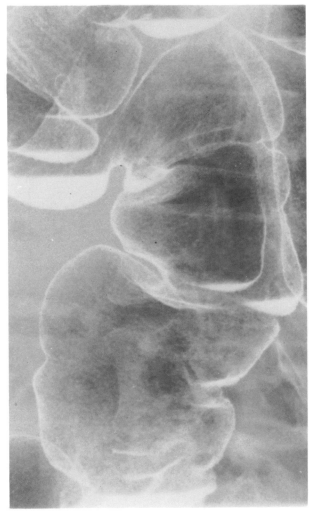

Fig. 5.6 Moderate ulcerative colitis shown by a double-contrast barium enema. Multiple small ulcers are visible with a granular appearance.

lost and the colon becomes shortened and narrowed (Fig. 5.8). Post-inflammatory polyps (pseudo-polyps) are often seen (Fig. 5.9) but usually spare the rectum. They are another feature of long-standing disease but may occur after the first attack and can occasionally regress.

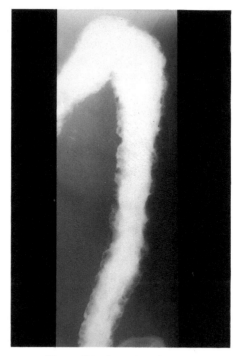

Fig. 5.7   Single-contrast ('instant') barium enema in a patient with severe ulcerative colitis. Deep ulceration is visible in the descending and distal transverse colon.

Colonoscopy

Colonoscopy is not necessary for the diagnosis of ulcerative colitis provided a good-quality barium enema is available and sigmoidoscopy with rectal biopsy has been performed. It is useful, however, if the barium X-ray is equivocal or normal, or if there is doubt concerning the differential diagnosis. The disease is often more extensive at colonoscopy than indicated radiologically. Multiple biopsies should be taken at sites from around the whole colon because, even if the mucosa appears to be macroscopically normal, histological assessment may reveal acute and/or chronic inflammatory changes. Colonoscopy is essential for the assessment of strictures and for cancer surveillance in those patients who have long-standing colitis (see Ch. 9).

Rectal histology

A rectal biopsy specimen should always be taken at the initial sigmoidoscopic examination (Fig. 1.2). The histological appearance may help to differentiate the appearances of Crohn's disease or infective colitis, or reveal changes of dysplasia (see Ch. 9).

Biopsy should be performed below 10 cm, i.e. below the peritoneal reflection, and from the posterior wall of the rectum. If this procedure is followed the risk of perforation is extremely small, especially if modern biopsy forceps are used (e.g. St Mark's biopsy forceps, KeyMed). The risk of significant haemorrhage is also minimal if small cup forceps are used.

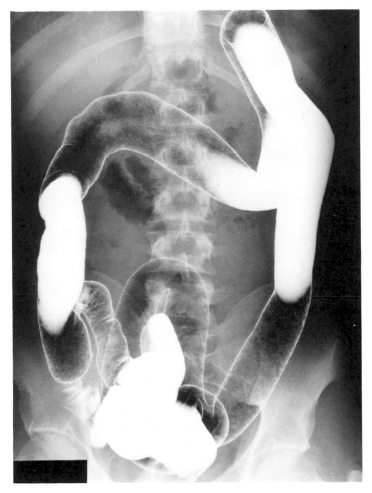

Fig. 5.8 Double-contrast barium enema in a patient with long-standing ulcerative colitis. The colon is narrowed and has lost the normal haustral pattern. The mucosa is granular, suggesting mildly active disease.

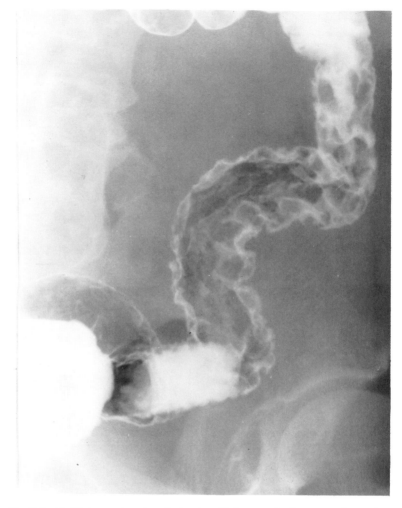

Fig. 5.9 Multiple pseudo-polyps in the sigmoid shown on barium enema in a patient with long-standing ulcerative colitis.

Differential diagnosis

The more common diagnoses that must be considered in patients with suspected ulcerative colitis are shown in Table 5.1. In patients with a short history of an acute onset of bloody diarrhoea, particularly those who have coexisting abdominal pain, an infective cause should always be vigorously excluded. However, patients with

Table 5.1   Differential diagnosis of ulcerative colitis

Disease	Clinical features	Sigmoidoscopic appearances	Features on barium enema
Ulcerative colitis	Blood and mucus predominant. Severe abdominal pain unusual	Diffuse inflammation involving rectum	Rectum always involved. Fine ulceration. Enema may be normal
Crohn's disease	Systemic upset, e.g. weight loss, fever common. Anal lesions and extracolonic involvement is frequently found	May be normal or patchy inflammation with aphthous or deep ulcers present	Segmental disease. Stricture or deep ulcers
Ischaemic colitis	Elderly patients sudden onset of symptoms. Pain and bleeding often predominant	Usually normal. Blood from above	Splenic flexure usually involved. Mucosal oedema predominant. Rectal involvement very rare
Infective	Sudden-onset fever common. Abdominal pain may predominate. Pathogens present in stool	Mild reddening of mucosa. Small ulcers rarely seen. Often indistinguishable from ulcerative colitis	Usually normal
Pseudo-membranous colitis	Recent history of antibiotic ingestion. *Clostridium difficile* present in stool	Pseudo-membrane or plaques overlying the mucosa	Discrete ulcers not seen
Amoebic colitis	History of travel in endemic area. Amoebae present in stool	Deep ulcers with normal surrounding mucosa	Discrete ulcers present. Amoeboma or strictures occur

underlying ulcerative colitis can present with an acute infective episode. The rectal histology is particularly helpful in the diagnosis of such patients. The presence of amoebae or schistosomal ova must be excluded in the biopsy specimens if the patient has recently been in endemic areas.

Sexually transmitted diseases can cause a proctitis in homosexual patients. Gonococcal proctitis can usually be distinguished sigmoidoscopically from ulcerative colitis since there are usually large quantities of purulent exudate covering the rectal mucosa. The diagnosis is made by culture. Chlamydia may also cause a proctitis. In patients with human immunodeficiency virus (HIV) infection, cytomegalovirus, herpes simplex, *Mycobacterium avium intracellulare* and Kaposi's sarcoma can all affect the colon.

INVESTIGATION OF CROHN'S DISEASE

Stool examination

The stool appearances in Crohn's disease are even more variable than those of ulcerative colitis because appearance is dependent upon the site and extent of the diseased bowel. The changes described for ulcerative colitis may also be observed in patients with Crohn's disease who have predominant colonic involvement, although bleeding is less common. Patients with extensive small bowel disease may have steatorrhoea, whereas watery, bile salt-induced diarrhoea may occur in patients with terminal ileal disease.

Laboratory investigations

Unlike patients with ulcerative colitis, most symptomatic patients with Crohn's disease will have abnormal laboratory indices at presentation. Such patients are often anaemic. The anaemia may be due to deficiencies of iron, vitamin B_{12} (in terminal ileal disease) or folate. Some patients with long-standing active disease will exhibit the anaemia of chronic disease due to suppression of erythropoiesis. Elevations of ESR and acute-phase reactants, such as C-reactive protein and orosomucoid, are often found in Crohn's disease and may be used as markers of disease activity. However, normal values for ESR are found in some patients who have active Crohn's disease. Raised platelet counts also reflect disease activity and may play a role in the increased thrombotic tendency in patients with active Crohn's disease. Serum albumin levels are useful because they reflect the degree of inflammation in the gut.

Sigmoidoscopy

Rectal examination prior to sigmoidoscopy may reveal the characteristic changes of perianal disease, with fleshy skin tags and fistulae

(Figs 4.1 and 4.2). The sigmoidoscopic appearances are variable: normal mucosa, patchy inflammation, aphthous ulceration (Fig. 5.10), deep ulceration or diffuse colitis may be seen. Even if the mucosa appears to be normal, a rectal biopsy should be taken because granulomas can be found on histological examination in some patients.

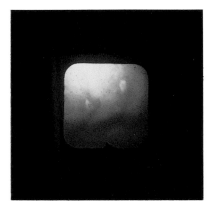

Fig. 5.10   Endoscopic appearances of aphthoid ulcers in the rectum of a patient with Crohn's disease.

Radiology

The small bowel enema (enteroclysis) has become the procedure of choice for the diagnosis of small intestinal Crohn's disease. The commonest appearances are thickening of the valvulae conniventes, oedema of the wall, and fissure ulcers; the latter two findings may give rise to the 'cobblestone' appearance (Figs 5.11 and 5.12). The lumen may be narrowed and there may be one or more strictures (Fig. 5.13). If these are sufficiently severe to cause obstruction, there may be proximal dilatation of the small bowel. Scattered aphthoid ulcers throughout the small intestine are not an uncommon finding and are only detected by a small bowel enema and are not seen with a barium meal and follow-through. Likewise the presence of fistulae, especially if multiple and complex, are also much better seen on a small bowel enema.

A double-contrast barium enema examination of the colon may show segmental involvement with superficial or deep ulcers (Fig. 5.14). Strictures may also occur in the colon (Fig. 5.15). The rectum, unlike that in ulcerative colitis, is frequently spared. In

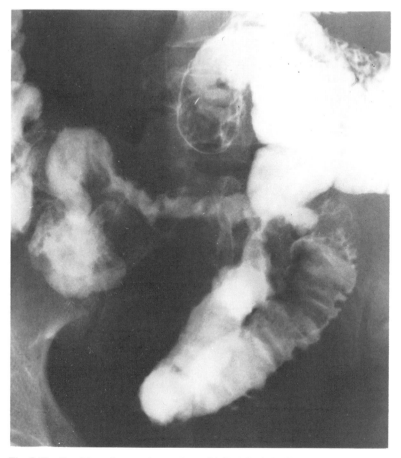

Fig. 5.11   Small bowel enema in a patient with ileal Crohn's disease. There is a long segment of disease in the terminal ileum, which is narrowed with mucosal oedema and fissure ulcers.

some patients, however, it can be impossible to differentiate between ulcerative colitis and Crohn's disease by the radiological appearances alone.

Indium-111 autologous neutrophil scanning

The principle of this technique is that autologous neutrophils are labelled with indium-111 (^{111}In) or technetium-99 and reinjected into the patient's circulation. The migration of the neutrophils into areas of focal inflammation can be detected by a gamma-counter scan

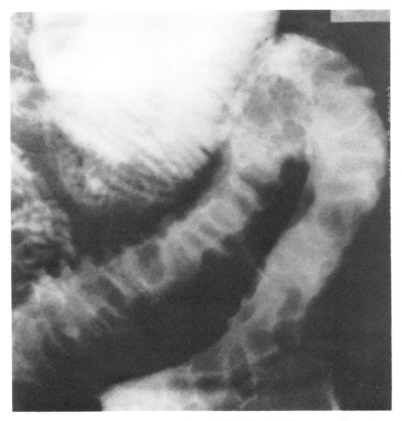

Fig. 5.12   Small bowel enema in a patient with ileal Crohn's disease — enlarged view. There is marked cobblestoning caused by mucosal oedema with fissure ulcers.

obtained 4 h after injection. Assessments of disease activity can be made, comparing the intensity of radionuclide uptake in eight segments of colon with the intensity of uptake by bone marrow, liver and spleen (Fig. 5.16). Results from this technique have correlated well with other parameters of activity. In addition, the four-day faecal white cell excretion of ^{111}In has also been shown to correlate closely with other markers of disease activity.

The advantage of the ^{111}In-labelled neutrophil technique is that, in addition to assessing the severity of disease, the site of disease can be localized, irrespective of previous surgical resections and the presence of an ileostomy or colostomy. The disadvantage is that the patients receive a radiation dose comparable to that of a barium

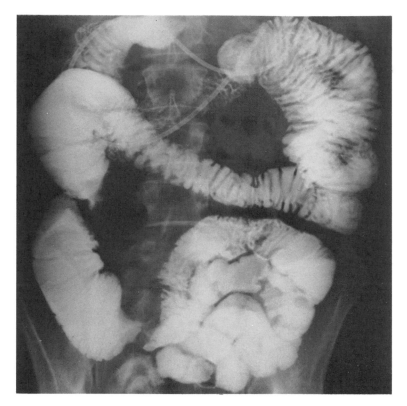

Fig. 5.13 Small bowel enema in a patient with Crohn's disease. At least two strictures are visible with a dilated segment of ileum between them.

enema examination, making repeated scanning undesirable, particularly in patients with Crohn's disease, who are often young. In addition, faecal collection is inconvenient. Thus, ^{111}In-scanning may have a role in difficult cases as a research tool but it is probably not necessarily indicated for the routine assessment of activity or extent of Crohn's disease.

Colonoscopy

Colonoscopy is particularly useful in assessing Crohn's disease. If unequivocal changes are seen on a double-contrast barium enema it is not always necessary to perform colonoscopy. However, it is valuable whenever there are problems in the diagnosis and/or the extent of colonic disease. In addition, skilled colonoscopists can

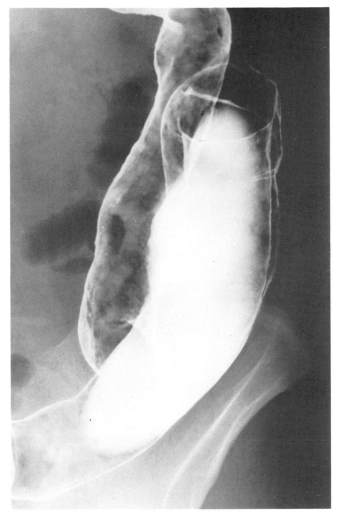

Fig. 5.14 Double-contrast barium enema showing aphthoid ulcers of Crohn's disease throughout the left colon.

often examine the terminal ileum, providing useful visual and histological information.

The appearances of Crohn's disease vary from scattered aphthoid ulcers (Fig. 17) to severe ulceration, which may be deep, punched-out ulcers or serpiginous (Figs 5.17 and 5.18). The inflammatory change is often focal and segmental in contrast to the diffuse, continuous inflammation of ulcerative colitis.

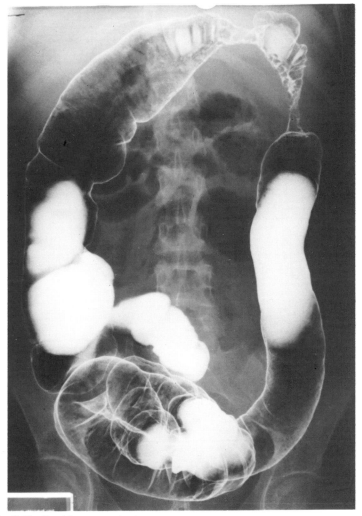

Fig. 5.15 Double-contrast barium enema in a patient with colonic Crohn's disease. There is stricturing at the splenic flexure, with aphthoid ulcers present just proximal to this as well as in the sigmoid colon. The patient also had multiple strictures in the small intestine, which is suggested by the loops of distended ileum.

Rectal histology

Rectal histology should always be examined in patients with suspected Crohn's disease. Epithelioid granulomas can be found in a rectal biopsy specimen in approximately 25% of patients with Crohn's disease. In addition, there are other changes which, if present, may help to distinguish Crohn's disease from other causes of inflammation. These changes include alterations in the mucosal pattern, irregular enlarged glands filled with exudate, and patchy mucosal inflammation without marked loss of goblet cell mucus.

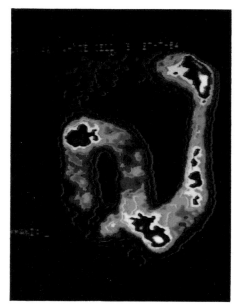

Fig. 5.16 An indium-labelled granulocyte scan in a patient with colonic Crohn's disease. There is uptake in the sigmoid, descending colon and splenic flexure but with little activity in the rectum.

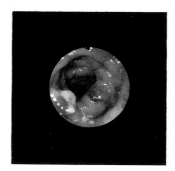

Fig. 5.17 Colonoscopic appearances of Crohn's disease in the transverse colon. The mucosal folds are thickened, irregular and friable. There are multiple small ulcers and a muco-purulent exudate.

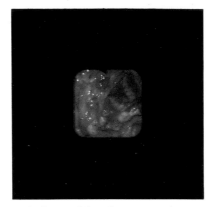

Fig. 5.18 Severe Crohn's disease of the colon seen at colonoscopy. There is deep, serpiginous ulceration with considerable mucosal thickening and an early 'cobblestone' pattern.

Differential diagnosis

In Caucasian patients, the main differential diagnosis is from ulcerative colitis and the other more common forms of colitis listed in Table 5.1. However, in non-Caucasian patients, it can be very difficult to distinguish the clinical and radiological features of Crohn's disease from those of ileocaecal tuberculosis. At presentation for patients with predominant oral and perineal ulceration, the diagnosis of Behçet's disease should be considered, although Behçet's disease is very uncommon in Western countries. Behçet's ulcers involving the gastrointestinal tract tend to be deeper and more punched out, although the mucosal changes can closely resemble those of Crohn's disease. Infections such as *Yersinia* may present as an acute terminal ileitis, which is often difficult to distinguish from acute Crohn's disease, even at operation. Stool culture and serology are helpful to exclude *Yersinia* infections.

FURTHER READING

Baron J H, Connell A M, Lennard-Jones J E 1964 Variation between observers in describing mucosal appearances in protocolitis. Br Med J i: 89–92

Bartram C 1976 Plain abdominal X-ray in acute colitis. Proc R Soc Med 67: 617–618

Nolan D J, Gupta R 1987 Modern imaging techniques for inflammatory bowel disease. In: Lee E C G (ed) Surgery of inflammatory bowel disorders. Churchill Livingstone, Edinburgh, pp 8–19

Pera A, Bellando P, Caldera D et al 1987 Colonoscopy in inflammatory bowel disease. Gastroenterology 92: 181–185

Surawicz C M, Belic L Rectal biopsy helps to distinguish acute self-limited colitis from idiopathic inflammatory bowel disease. Gastroenterology 86: 104–113

6 Extraintestinal manifestations of inflammatory bowel disease

Approximately one-third of all patients with ulcerative colitis and Crohn's disease will suffer from at least one of the wide spectrum of extraintestinal manifestations. In a minority of patients they are the presenting clinical feature and, rarely, they may precede symptoms referable to gastrointestinal disease.

Extraintestinal manifestations may be classified as:

1. Associated with active disease. For Crohn's disease, this implies active colonic disease for the majority of patients with acute skin, eye or joint disease.
2. Unassociated with disease activity.
3. Complications of small intestinal disease or resection.

THE SKIN

The most important cutaneous manifestations are erythema nodosum and pyoderma gangrenosum (Fig. 6.1). Although the reported incidence varies, about 2–10% of patients with ulcerative colitis or Crohn's colitis will develop one of these troublesome skin lesions. The aetiology of these lesions remains obscure. The eruption of the red nodules of erythema nodosum on the shins, thighs and arms indicates coexisting active colonic inflammation. Treatment of the colonic inflammation with corticosteroids or surgery usually results in a rapid clinical improvement. Pyoderma gangrenosum usually presents initially as pustules (which are sterile on culture) which gradually enlarge, coalesce and ulcerate (Figs 6.1 and 6.2). It is rare but occurs more often with ulcerative colitis than Crohn's disease. Pyoderma is generally more resistant to medical therapy than erythema nodosum and colectomy may be required to control the skin lesion.

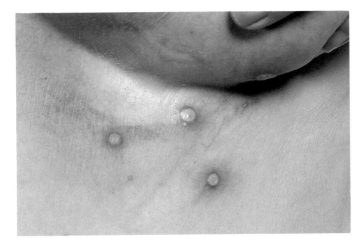

Fig. 6.1   Early lesions of pyoderma gangrenosum.

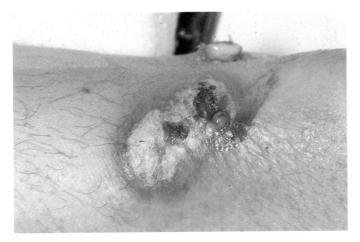

Fig. 6.2   Pyoderma gangrenosum — the early lesions have coalesced and ulcerated.

THE JOINTS

There are two types of arthritis occurring in association with ulcerative colitis or Crohn's disease. In the first, an asymmetrical transient non-deforming arthropathy occurs in association with active intestinal inflammation. Although any joint may be inflamed, the large joints of the lower extremities are most commonly involved. The joint becomes hot, swollen and tender. Treatment is aimed at controlling the active colitis; non-steroidal anti-inflammatory agents may be required for symptomatic relief of the arthropathy but should be avoided if possible as they may aggravate the colitis.

The second form of arthritis that occurs is sacroiliitis and ankylosing spondylitis (Fig. 6.3). There is a close association between ankylosing spondylitis and HLA-B27, although in contrast to patients with sporadic ankylosing spondylitis who are 90% positive for HLA-B27, patients with ulcerative colitis and Crohn's disease have a lower incidence of 75%. The clinical course of the spondylitis is independent of the severity, extent or duration of the inflammatory bowel disease. Treatment involves non-steroidal anti-inflammatory drugs and physiotherapy. Sacroiliitis may be asymptomatic but can be a cause of back pain. It does not progress to ankylosing spondylitis and is not associated with HLA-B27.

The relationship between mucosal inflammation and arthropathy is not clear. It has been proposed that the inflamed bowel leads to increased mucosal permeability, which in turn allows exposure to

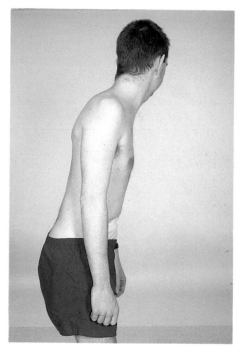

Fig. 6.3   Ankylosing spondylitis in a patient with ulcerative colitis.

enteric bacterial antigens that may be important in the pathogenesis of the arthropathy.

THE EYES

The most commonly occurring ocular lesions in association with either ulcerative colitis or Crohn's disease, in order of frequency of occurrence, are anterior uveitis, episcleritis (Fig. 6.4) and conjunctivitis. The reported frequency of eye lesions varies from approximately 3% to 14% of all cases of inflammatory bowel disease. Although it is often associated with active mucosal inflammation, uveitis can precede the onset of gastrointestinal symptoms or may occur after intestinal resection. Uveitis usually responds to local and systemic corticosteroid therapy. The explanation for the association with inflammatory bowel disease is not known. It has been suggested that circulating immune complexes may play a role in the pathogenesis of the eye lesions, but there is little evidence to support this hypothesis.

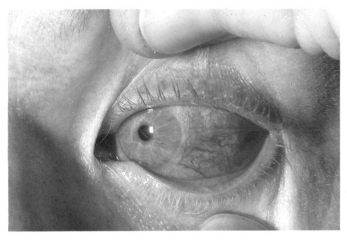

Fig. 6.4   Episcleritis in a patient with active ulcerative colitis.

HEPATOBILIARY MANIFESTATIONS

Since the first description in 1872 of fatty liver occurring in a young man with ulceration of the colon, several hepatobiliary conditions have been reported in association with ulcerative colitis and Crohn's disease. A list of these conditions is shown in Table 6.1.

Table 6.1   Hepatobiliary conditions found in association with inflammatory bowel disease

---

Biliary
Primary sclerosing cholangitis
Cholangiocarcinoma
Primary biliary cirrhosis
Gallstones[1]

Hepatocellular
Fatty liver
Chronic active hepatitis
Cirrhosis
Hepatoma

Miscellaneous
Granulomas
Amyloidosis
Liver abscess
Drug reactions, e.g. sulphasalazine

---

[1] Only in Crohn's disease.

Approximately 50% of patients with active inflammatory bowel disease may have minor abnormalities of hepatic function. Significant liver disease occurs in 5–10%. The commonest abnormality is fatty liver, which is usually seen in patients with severe attacks of ulcerative colitis or Crohn's disease, particularly in those who are malnourished and receiving corticosteroid therapy. A markedly increased prevalence of cholesterol gallstones is found in patients with Crohn's disease involving the terminal ileum because of a decrease in bile acid absorption. This interruption in the normal enterohepatic circulation causes the bile to become supersaturated with cholesterol, leading to the formation of cholesterol gallstones. Patients with Crohn's disease who do not have terminal ileal involvement, and patients with ulcerative colitis, have a normal prevalence of gallstones when compared with control subjects.

Several hepatobiliary disorders have been described in association with ulcerative colitis and, less commonly, in Crohn's disease. Until recently, these were considered to be separate entities. Over the last decade, however, it has become clear that the disorders of pericholangitis, chronic active hepatitis, and primary sclerosing cholangitis and cholangiocarcinoma all represent part of a spectrum of one hepatobiliary disorder, namely primary sclerosing cholangitis. Primary sclerosing cholangitis is characterized by an intense inflammatory fibrosis involving the biliary system, which results in stricturing and dilatation of the bile ducts. The whole biliary system is usually affected but the changes may be localized to either predominant intrahepatic or extrahepatic involvement.

The diagnosis of primary sclerosing cholangitis is based on the cholangiographic demonstration of beading and stricturing of the biliary system, usually by the endoscopic technique (Fig. 6.5). Liver biopsy is also helpful, but the changes seen histologically may be patchy and in the majority of cases they are not diagnostic. Biochemical screening usually reveals a cholestatic pattern; marked elevation of the serum alkaline phosphatase is the earliest and predominant abnormality. The aetiology of primary sclerosing cholangitis is not known. Current evidence suggests that immunological

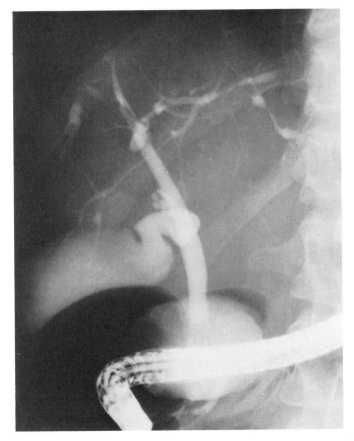

Fig. 6.5 An endoscopic retrograde cholangiogram of a patient with ulcerative colitis and primary sclerosing cholangitis. The intrahepatic bile ducts are irregular, with characteristic beading and stricturing.

mechanisms are important in the bile duct damage, perhaps triggered by enteric organisms in susceptible patients.

There is an increased incidence (10- to 20-fold increase) of cholangiocarcinoma in patients with ulcerative colitis. Patients with primary sclerosing cholangitis also develop bile duct carcinoma and it is probable that all patients with ulcerative colitis and cholangiocarcinoma have an underlying primary sclerosing cholangitis.

AMYLOIDOSIS

Amyloidosis is rare and is mostly associated with Crohn's disease. It has the characteristics of secondary amyloid (AA) and tends to involve the liver, kidney, spleen and other organs, including the intestine. The condition is usually irreversible and may be fatal as a result of hepatic or renal failure. However, it may regress following surgical resection of the Crohn's disease.

VASCULAR MANIFESTATIONS

Thromboembolic disease is an important extraintestinal complication of active ulcerative colitis and active Crohn's disease. It occurs in about 5–10% of patients and is an important cause of death in a minority of them. The reason for the hypercoagulable state is multifactorial and is due to a combination of high platelet count, increased fibrinogen and factor VIII levels, and activation of other factors.

MISCELLANEOUS CONDITIONS

Nephrolithiasis occurs in about 2–10% of patients with Crohn's disease. The most common type of kidney stone is that formed of uric acid. Calcium oxalate stones are the next most common and result from hyperoxaluria, which may be associated with ileal Crohn's disease.

FURTHER READING

Chapman R W 1991 Aetiology and natural history of primary sclerosing cholangitis: a decade of progress? Gut 32: 1433–1435

Snook J A 1990 Extra-intestinal manifestations of Crohn's disease. In: Jewell D P, Snook J A (eds) Topics in gastroenterology 17. Blackwell Scientific Publications, Oxford, pp 175–186

7 Medical management

ULCERATIVE COLITIS

Ulcerative colitis, unlike Crohn's disease, can be cured by removing the colon. However, the majority of patients with ulcerative colitis can be managed medically throughout their lives without resorting to surgery. The disease is characterized by acute exacerbations punctuating variable periods of remission. The aim of medical treatment is twofold: to treat acute attacks effectively and to maintain remission.

Treatment of the acute attack

The treatment of acute ulcerative colitis depends on the severity of the attack and the extent of the colon involved in the disease. The classic controlled clinical studies performed in Oxford in the late 1950s by Truelove established the benefit of corticosteroids in acute ulcerative colitis; corticosteroids still provide the mainstay of acute therapy. They may be administered topically, orally or intravenously; the route chosen depends upon the severity and extent of the inflammation (Ch. 4). Several different steroid formulations can be administered rectally (Table 7.1). Different preparations can be tried according to individual patient preference.

Proctitis

For patients with disease limited to the rectum (i.e. the sigmoidoscope can be passed beyond the proximal limit of the inflammation) a topical steroid preparation or a suppository are the most convenient preparations. Patients are often given sulphasalazine orally in addition. Unfortunately, proctitis can often be difficult to heal.

Table 7.1 Commonly used topical steroid preparations in the treatment of acute ulcerative colitis

Generic name	Trade name	Steroid dose/ enema insertion	Comment
Prednisolone phosphate	Predsol enema	20 mg	Well absorbed rectally
Prednisolone metasulpho- benzoate	Predenema	20 mg	Poorly absorbed
Prednisolone metasulpho- benzoate (in aerosol pack)	Predfoam	20 mg	Easier to retain, particularly in elderly patients
Hydrocortisone (in viscous suspension)	Cortenema	100 mg	Well absorbed
Hydrocortisone acetate (in aerosol pack)	Colifoam	100 mg	Well absorbed, easier to retain
Prednisolone phosphate	Predsol suppositories	5 mg/ suppository	Used for proctitis only

If topical corticosteroids fail, sulphasalazine enemas or suppositories or a 5-aminosalicylic acid (5-ASA) enema can be tried. Many of these patients show severe constipation in the proximal colon and may feel better if this is cleared. If there is still no response, oral corticosteroids should be given, and in some patients symptoms are sufficiently severe to warrant intravenous therapy in hospital. Occasionally, a severe proctitis causes sufficient symptoms, despite maximal therapy, to warrant surgical resection.

Mild attacks

Mild attacks are those in which patients are only passing four to five motions daily, usually with blood or mucus, but who remain systemically well. They should be treated with oral prednisolone 20 mg daily for a period of four weeks, together with a corticosteroid retention enema or foam preparation. If remission occurs, the steroids can be tailed off. If symptoms do not settle, the steriod dose should be increased.

Moderate attacks

Moderate attacks are those where the patient is passing six or more motions daily but, again, without evidence of systemic illness. They should be given 40 mg prednisolone daily for the first week, 30 mg daily for the second week, and then 20 mg daily for the subsequent four weeks before the steroids are tailed off. Topical steroids should also be given. If the disease does not settle, patients should be treated as for a severe attack.

Severe attacks

Patients with severe attacks of ulcerative colitis should be admitted to hospital for monitoring of pulse rate, blood pressure, temperature and signs of colonic dilatation or perforation. Daily management decisions are made jointly by physician and surgeon. Plain abdominal X-rays should be obtained daily until the symptoms have settled. Intravenous fluids and blood transfusions are given to correct electrolyte disturbances and anaemia, together with intravenous prednisolone (60 mg per day) or hydrocortisone (400 mg daily). Antibiotics are not indicated unless a specific infection is present. A rectal drip of hydrocortisone (100 mg in 100 ml) is administered twice daily. Opinions differ as to whether, in a severe attack, patients should be nil by mouth or allowed food. However, there is no firm evidence that stopping oral food intake influences the outcome, although many patients are nauseated and anorectic and prefer to avoid food. Approximately 70% of patients will respond to this intensive intravenous and rectal steroid regimen after five to seven days. These patients should be commenced on oral prednisolone therapy (40 mg per day) and oral sulphasalazine or its equivalent. The prednisolone is then tailed off over the next six weeks. Patients who do not respond to this regimen or who deteriorate during therapy should be considered for urgent colectomy, preferably by an experienced colorectal surgeon (see Ch. 8). Acute colonic dilatation at presentation is not an indication for immediate surgery, but if the colonic diameter has not decreased after 24 h then colectomy should be carried out. However, surgery must not be delayed if the dilatation occurs during the treatment period.

Refractory colitis

Some patients either relapse quickly after stopping corticosteroids or are slow to settle and develop chronic grumbling symptoms. If the patient has a proctitis or left-sided colitis, a plain abdominal X-ray should be taken to determine whether there is proximal constipation. This is present surprisingly frequently and should be relieved by gentle purgation (e.g., oral Picolax or Golytely). Relief of the constipation often allows the disease to settle.

If the chronic, continuous symptoms continue, immunosuppressives can be added to the corticosteroids, e.g. azathioprine 2.0–2.5 mg/kg body weight. Patients receiving azathioprine should have regular blood counts. High-dose corticosteroids, given on alternate days, is another stratagem which is occasionally successful for patients with chronically active disease and may allow the inflammation to settle without inducing too many side effects.

Maintenance of remission

The major use of sulphasalazine is in long-term maintenance therapy. Controlled clinical trials have shown that continuous administration of oral sulphasalazine reduces the frequency of recurrent attacks over a period of many years. The optimal dose for a maximal clinical effect with the least side effects is 2 g daily. Sulphasalazine consists of 5-ASA (the active moiety) linked to a sulphapyridine molecule by an azo bond. The drug is poorly absorbed in the small intestine and the majority of an orally administered dose passes into the colon. Once in the colon, bacteria cleave the azo bond and release the two individual moieties.

The mode of action of sulphasalazine is not known. The drug is well tolerated by the majority of patients with ulcerative colitis. However, there are a number of dose-related and non-dose-related side effects, which are shown in Table 7.2. The dose-related side effects of sulphasalazine can often be overcome by starting at a reduced dose of 0.5 g per day and gradually increasing to the full therapeutic dose of 2 g per day.

The active moiety of sulphasalazine is 5-ASA, whereas the sulphapyridine moiety mediates the majority of the adverse reactions. Hence several new preparations of 5-ASA have been developed which provide high concentrations of the drug in the colon (5-ASA cannot be given orally in a simple preparation because it is rapidly absorbed in the small intestine and excreted in the urine leading to high systemic concentrations but low concentrations in the colonic lumen). The generic name for 5-ASA is mesalazine and it is now available either in an enteric-coated form (Asacol) or as a slow-release preparation (Pentasa). Both preparations allow release of the 5-ASA once the luminal pH becomes 7.0 or more.

Table 7.2 The side effects of sulphasalazine

Dose-related	Non-dose-related
Nausea	Skin rashes (+ Stevens-Johnson syndrome)
Vomiting	Erythema nodosum
Diarrhoea	Heinz body haemolytic anaemia
Headache	Folate deficiency
Male infertility (reversible)	Agranulocytosis

Asacol consists of 5-ASA coated with the resin, Eudragit-S, which is pH sensitive whereas Pentasa consists of micro granules of 5-ASA coated with a semi-permeable membrane. Pentasa may release the 5-ASA rather more gradually than Asacol once the surrounding pH rises to 7.0. An alternative approach has been to couple two molecules of 5-ASA together via an azo bond. This compound is olsalazine, which has similar pharmacodynamics to sulphasalazine and gives high concentrations of 5-ASA in the colonic lumen. Olsalazine has recently been shown, in an open study, to be more effective than mesalazine at reducing the relapse rate.

All of these new drugs are equally as effective as sulphasalazine but are associated with fewer side effects. If olsalazine is used, the dose must be built up gradually and the drug taken with food in order to avoid loosening of stool. If Asacol is used, the serum creatinine should be checked regularly as some cases of renal failure have been reported on this drug. Since they are more expensive than sulphasalazine, they should be used primarily in patients known to be intolerant to sulphasalazine, those who are sulphonamide sensitive, and in young men who wish to have a family. This latter group may develop infertility on sulphasalazine, although this is readily reversible on stopping the drug. However, as the male infertility is mediated by the sulphonamide moiety, it does not occur with the 5-ASA preparations.

CROHN'S DISEASE

The management of patients with active Crohn's disease owes as much to art as to science. The reasons for this lie in the unpredictable and variable nature of the disease: variation in the site and extent of macroscopic intestinal involvement; lack of correlation between symptoms and the amount of gut affected; and an inconsistent response to medical or surgical therapy. Unlike ulcerative colitis, Crohn's disease cannot be cured by surgery, because the disease usually recurs after resection in a previously uninvolved segment of gut (Ch. 9). The best way to manage Crohn's disease is to treat and control a current problem causing symptoms. Several different approaches can be tried. Drug treatment is only one aspect of therapy; other options include dietary manipulation, nutritional supplementation and surgery.

Before embarking on drug therapy, it is important to obtain a precise account of the patient's symptoms. In some instances, symptoms such as intermittent colicky abdominal pain and nausea will not be due to active bowel inflammation but due to complications of the disease, for example intestinal obstruction secondary to fibrous strictures. Watery diarrhoea in patients with terminal ileal disease, or in those who have had an ileal resection, may be secondary to bile salt malabsorption. In addition to the clinical assessment, endoscopic and radiological investigations should be used to assess the site, extent and complications of the disease. Potential nutritional deficiences such as vitamin B_{12} and iron deficiency should be excluded. Once this process of assessment is complete, an appropriate management strategy should be decided for each individual patient by both the physician and the surgeon.

Drug treatment

In contrast to its use in ulcerative colitis, maintenance therapy with sulphasalazine has not been shown to be effective in reducing the relapse rate of Crohn's disease, even following surgical excision of all macroscopic disease. However, sulphasalazine is effective for the treatment of active colonic disease although it seems to be much less useful in treating small bowel disease.

As in ulcerative colitis, the main role of corticosteroids is to suppress acute inflammation in the involved segment of the gut. Mild to moderate exacerbations should be treated with regimens similar to those described for ulcerative colitis. More severe cases are admitted to hospital and treated with 60 mg prednisolone or 400 mg hydrocortisone given intravenously for five to seven days before introducing a reducing dose of oral prednisolone. Patients should not be given corticosteroids long term because these agents do not prevent recurrent disease and it puts the patient at risk of complications such as osteoporosis. Patients who relapse quickly on steroid withdrawal should be considered for treatment with the immuno-suppressants azathioprine or 6-mercaptopurine. Immunosuppres-sives usually take several weeks to exert an effect and therefore, once started, it seems sensible to continue treatment for at least one year if response occurs. Cyclosporin (5 mg/kg) is currently being evaluated for Crohn's disease and may be beneficial for chronic, active or steroid-dependent disease.

Topical corticosteroids are reserved for the treatment of oral Crohn's disease, and disease of the distal colon and anus.

The antibiotic metronidazole may also be helpful in the treatment of Crohn's disease, particularly in those who have perianal disease. Metronidazole given for four months has been shown to be as effective as sulphasalazine for the treatment of active small bowel and colonic Crohn's disease. It is also indicated if there is bacterial overgrowth in the small intestine. The major side effect of metroni-dazole is peripheral neuropathy. This effect is dose related and usually reverses on lowering the dose or stopping the therapy.

Antidiarrhoeal agents, such as loperamide or codeine phosphate, may provide symptomatic relief but are not to be recommended for general use. The cause of the diarrhoea should be determined and appropriately treated. Bile-salt-induced diarrhoea may respond to cholestyramine.

The role of diet in treatment

The role of diet in the aetiology of Crohn's disease is discussed in Chapter 3. Over the last decade, there has been renewed interest in the manipulation of diet for the treatment of patients with Crohn's disease. The diet may be altered for one of the following reasons: nutritional support, primary treatment of active disease, and to prevent relapse or progression of the disease.

When severely malnourished patients with Crohn's disease are admitted to hospital, they may require intensive nutritional supple-mentation. This can be given by infusing nutritionally balanced liquid feeds using a fine-bore nasogastric tube. Although total parenteral nutrition is often used, it is seldom truly indicated. Its use should be reserved for a few well-defined situations: before and after surgery in malnourished patients; the 'short-bowel' syndrome; and high enterocutaneous fistulae.

Nutrition as primary treatment of active disease

In view of the possibility that certain undefined dietary antigens may play a role in the pathogenesis of Crohn's disease, elemental diets have been tried in patients with active Crohn's disease. The elemental diet consists of protein as amino acids, with a small amount of bi- and tripeptides, together with carbohydrate in the form of glucose; most essential micronutrients are also included. To obtain full nutrition, 3 litres per day are required. This volume can give rise to diarrhoea but this is minimized if given slowly through a nasogastric tube, e.g. overnight. Elemental diets have proved to be as effective as prednisolone when given over four weeks to patients with active Crohn's disease. The problems with this approach are those of poor patient compliance, relapse on stopping the diet, and expense. Combination therapy of prednisolone and an elemental diet has not been tested in controlled trials.

Nutrition to prevent relapse or progression of the disease

Initial studies suggested that a low-sugar, fibre-rich diet might be helpful in preventing relapse and disease progression. Unfortunately, a multicentre controlled trial found no significant difference in relapse rates in those patients who took a low-sugar, fibre-rich diet when compared with those who received their normal diet.

Food intolerance has also recently been studied by the use of elimination diets. However, the results of this approach are unconvincing and, at the present time, there is little place for dietary restriction.

Treatment of children

Ulcerative colitis and Crohn's disease in children should be treated in exactly the same way as in adults, apart from adjusting dosages of drugs. There is considerable reluctance to treat these diseases aggressively when they occur at a young age, especially in the use of corticosteroids. However, growth and development are more likely to be stunted by chronic, grumbling disease than by short courses of prednisolone when there is evidence of active inflammation. Diet is particularly important in maintaining growth and frequent assessments of intake should be made by a dietitian. However, for ulcerative colitis, the whole colon is affected in at least 50% of children. This is much higher than for adults, and so the overall colectomy rate tends to be high in these children.

Treatment during pregnancy

Although there may be a high rate of miscarriage if conception occurs while intestinal inflammation is active, there is no evidence that either ulcerative colitis or Crohn's disease affects a pregnancy, nor does the pregnancy have a deleterious effect on the disease. Sulphasalazine, corticosteroids and immunosuppressive agents should be used as indicated by the activity of the disease since there is minimal risk to the fetus from these drugs, but considerable risk to both the fetus and mother if the disease is not managed properly. Thus, for both diseases, treatment should be directed towards controlling active inflammation and maintaining remission using the regimens described earlier.

FURTHER READING

Jewell D P 1989 Corticosteroids for the management of ulcerative colitis and Crohn's disease. Gastroenterol Clin North Am 18: 21–23

Russell R I 1991 Dietary and nutritional management of Crohn's disease. Aliment Pharmacol Ther 5: 211–226

Thomson A B R 1991 New developments in the use of 5-aminosalicylic acid in patients with inflammatory bowel disease. Aliment Pharmacol Ther 5: 449–470

Willoughby C P 1990 Inflammatory bowel disease and pregnancy. In: Allan R N, Keighley M R B, Alexander-Williams J, Hawkins C F (eds) Inflammatory bowel diseases. Churchill Livingstone, Edinburgh, pp 547–558

8 Surgical treatment

ULCERATIVE COLITIS

The decision to perform surgery is a joint decision between the physician and specialist surgeon. The main indications for surgery in patients with ulcerative colitis are failed medical treatment, dysplasia or carcinoma, toxic dilatation, perforation or haemorrhage. There are now several surgical alternatives to be considered. Clinicians must be aware of these choices and be prepared to give a fair account of the advantages and disadvantages of each in discussion with their patients.

Proctocolectomy and ileostomy

The operation of proctocolectomy has played an important role in the development of surgery for ulcerative colitis over the last 25 years and is still the procedure favoured by many surgeons. The reasons for this are fourfold: it removes all the diseased tissue in one operation; it disposes of any cancer risk; it is a well-tried and usually uncomplicated technique; and the patient is able to return home and to work as soon as possible.

Recent improvements in operative technique which include a close rectal dissection and an intersphincteric excision of the anus have reduced the incidence of damage to pelvic nerves and delayed perineal wound healing. The major drawback associated with the procedure is the resulting ileostomy: although many patients will accept and adapt to a stoma, there is a psychological and social cost.

Proctocolectomy is still the first choice for older patients coming to surgery and for patients with locally advanced rectal cancer complicating their colitis. Improvements in stoma care have considerably reduced the incidence of skin problems, leakage and ulcer; the help and advice of a stoma therapist are invaluable. Segmental resections for ulcerative colitis are never successful.

Kock continent ileostomy

A continent ileostomy may be indicated in patients who have already had a proctocolectomy and are unhappy with a conventional ileostomy. A complete continence rate of over 90% can be expected. The contraindications to this procedure are extensive small bowel resection, Crohn's disease, young age and old age. The anatomical arrangement of the pouch, nipple valve and low stoma site are shown in Figure 8.1. The construction of an ileostomy reservoir leads to bacterial colonization and morphological changes in the pouch mucosa, but there are no identifiable long-term nutritional sequelae. However, the introduction of another type of surgical alternative has meant that the Kock pouch will have only a limited place in the surgical management of colitis.

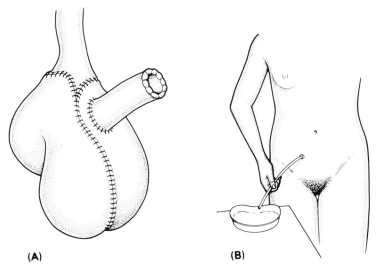

(A)   **(B)**

Fig. 8.1 Diagrammatic representations of the Kock pouch (**A**) and of a patient emptying the pouch with a catheter (**B**).

Ileorectal anastomosis

In those patients (usually only a small number) who have relative sparing of the rectum from colitis, an ileorectal anastomosis may be indicated (Fig. 8.2). For selected children especially, this may be an excellent option while they mature through adolescence. As there may be a relapse of colitis in the rectum with frequency and even incontinence, about 30% of patients will have to be converted to an

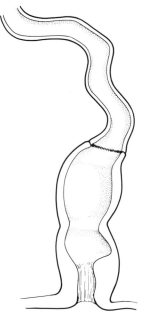

Fig. 8.2 An ileorectal anastomosis.

ileostomy. In the longer term, there is also a risk of malignant change in the rectal stump of about 3% of patients. Follow-up after an ileorectal anastomosis must be meticulous with annual flexible sigmoidoscopy and biopsy. Bowel function is usually good while rectal disease is quiescent, with three to four bowel actions per day on average.

Restorative proctocolectomy: the pouch operation

The new sphincter-saving operations have the advantage that they eradicate the disease and its cancer risk as effectively as a procto-colectomy, but they do not leave a perineal wound and make a stoma unnecessary.

In 1976, Parks and colleagues introduced the technique of a pelvic triple-loop or S-shaped ileal reservoir sewn to the anus after a mucosal proctectomy. Although about 50% of the early patients were unable to empty the reservoir spontaneously, technical modi-fications have resolved the problem.

The reservoir itself has been modified and the results of S- (three loops), J- (two loops) and W- (four loops) shaped reservoirs have been reported (Fig. 8.3).

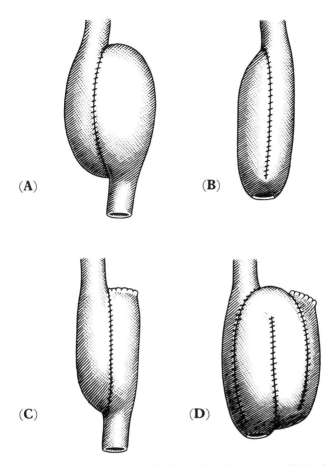

Fig. 8.3 Ileal reservoir designs: (**A**) the triplicated or S pouch; (**B**) the duplicated or J pouch; (**C**) the lateral or isoperistaltic pouch; (**D**) the four-loop or W pouch.

In all three types of this operation, the rectum is removed to the pelvic floor, preserving the anal sphincter. After carefully mobilizing the small bowel mesentery, a reservoir is fashioned and sewn down to the anus. The newly formed reservoir and ileoanal anastomosis are usually protected by a proximal loop ileostomy (Fig. 8.4), which is closed about eight weeks later.

The operation is suitable for motivated informed patients with ulcerative colitis who have not already had a proctocolectomy. Although age is not an absolute bar, patients under 60 years have the best functional results. Crohn's disease is a contraindication because active small bowel disease may result in pouch or anastomotic

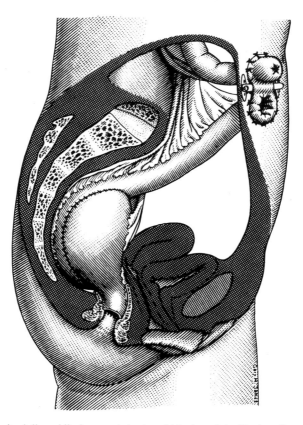

Fig. 8.4 A triplicated ileal reservoir in situ within the pelvis. The loop ileostomy can be closed through a peristomal incision eight weeks after the pouch operation.

failure. Construction of the pouch can be carried out at the same time as a total colectomy, but is usually protected with a loop ileostomy. A one-stage procedure can be done but would be unwise in those patients with severe colitis or in whom the diagnosis is not clearly established. Some patients with early malignant change can still have a pouch operation, but it would be contraindicated in patients who have an obvious rectal cancer. Although in the literature there are no recorded postoperative deaths, the early years following the introduction of the operation have not been without problems. The most frequent post-operative complication is pelvic sepsis, usually as a result of anal anastomotic dehiscence; this can give rise to prolonged infection which can occasionally require the removal of the pouch. 'Pouchitis' is a poorly understood complication, but it usually responds to metronidazole or Augmentin. A few patients may require topical corticosteroids or 5-ASA. Small bowel obstruction from adhesions and ileostomy dysfunction with dehydration and hyponatraemia from the proximally placed temporary loop stoma are also not uncommon. However, about 75% of patients do not have complications.

When the loop ileostomy is closed, about 10% of patients will have minor degrees of discharge or soiling, especially at night. Frank incontinence is unusual and pouch function improves over the first 12 months after ileostomy closure. Most patients have a normal sensation of pouch filling, and are able to defer evacuation without urgency.

Stool frequency will vary from three to six per day, and there is some evidence that the larger pouch volume of the W-shaped reservoir will give a lower stool frequency. As with a conventional ileostomy, the effluent is likely to become more solid but some patients continue to require codeine phosphate or loperamide.

Overall, only 5% of pouches have had to be removed for various reasons, including Crohn's disease, patient unsuitability or poor function. In a recent survey, 87% of patients favoured the pouch over an ileostomy for reasons that included confidence, cleanliness, sexual self-image, social and sporting activity, and ease of carrying out work.

The long-term functional results of the pelvic pouch have to be established. Although bacterial colonization and pouch ileal mucosal inflammation have been documented, these do not appear to correlate with function and no nutritional sequelae have been discovered. The early results of restorative proctocolectomy are so encouraging that the procedure should now gain widespread acceptance.

Emergency surgery

If an attack of ulcerative colitis is so severe or develops into a toxic dilatation, emergency surgery may be needed and can be life saving. At one time a proctocolectomy was advocated, removing all the disease in one stage. A pelvic dissection at the end of a careful and difficult colectomy avoiding perforation may increase morbidity, and with the advent of pouch procedures most surgeons now prefer a subtotal colectomy with ileostomy and mucous fistula or similar variant. This is a shorter, safer procedure and allows for easier identification of the rectal stump and dissection at the subsequent restorative proctectomy with a pouch.

CROHN'S DISEASE

The underlying philosophy of surgery for Crohn's disease is different from that for ulcerative colitis. As Crohn's disease is a diffuse and discontinuous disease of the gastrointestinal tract, it cannot be cured by surgery.

Consequently, surgery is reserved for the complications of Crohn's disease for which there will be several absolute and relative indications (Table 8.1). The basis of the surgical approach is conservation and, as there will be some debate about these indications, patients are best managed using a joint approach between physician and surgeon — not only will patients be on steroids and immunosuppressants but a high proportion will develop a recurrence in time. The surgical approach now adopted, therefore, is one of limited excision of macroscopic disease, which is less likely to result in patients with short gut syndrome.

Table 8.1   Indications for surgery in Crohn's disease

Absolute
Free perforation
Massive haemorrhage
Possible appendicitis
Carcinoma

Relative
Recurrent obstruction
Chronic obstruction
Malabsorption
Intra-abdominal abscess
Toxic megacolon
Retarded growth
Ureteric obstruction

Optional/occasional
Perianal fistula/abscess
Intra-abdominal fistula
Blind loop syndrome
Anorectal incontinence
Rectovaginal fistula
Enterovesical fistula
Abdominal wall fistula
Colonic stricture
Dyspareunia
Abdominal mass

Small bowel disease

Resection

The classic Crohn's lesion involving the terminal 10–20 cm of the ileum with its characteristic thickened pipe-like appearance is best treated by resection. This is sometimes called a limited right hemicolectomy, and a section of caecum and appendix is removed with the specimen, the ileum being joined to the ascending colon with a straight ileocolic anastomosis.

Minimal surgery

In more complicated cases, in whom a number of skip lesions are present, wide resections will result in multiple anastomoses and a short gut syndrome. Here, mini-resections or strictureplasties are the best option. Strictureplasty (Fig. 8.5) can be safely carried out

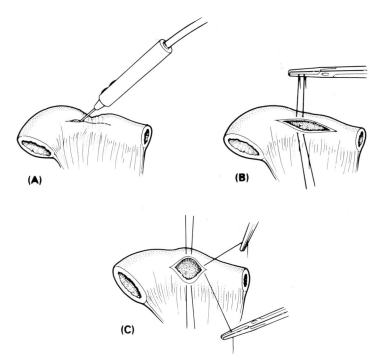

Fig. 8.5 Diagram to show the stages of a strictureplasty: (**A**) longitudinal incision across the stenosis using cutting diathermy; (**B**) incision completed across the stenosis from normal proximal to normal distal bowel; (**C**) stay sutures provide lateral traction. A central mattress suture approximates the two ends of the incision.

through involved ileum, but it is important to characterize the whole of the small intestine so that a distal obstruction is not overlooked. Multiple procedures involving ten or more strictures can be safely achieved during a single operation.

Enterocutaneous fistula

Patients with enterocutaneous fistulae have complicated problems and will often be malnourished, hyponatraemic and septic. Skin involvement can be a major challenge to a stoma therapist. Where there is a complicated fistula, abscesses must be drained and a proximal defunctioning stoma may be life saving. When sepsis has been abolished and the patient restored to a good nutritional state, the fistula and involved bowel can be resected and the bowel re-anastomosed. In post-operative fistulae in which there is neither evidence of underlying macroscopic disease nor evidence of distal obstruction, there should be spontaneous healing.

Duodenal disease

This is rare but wherever possible it should be managed by stric-tureplasty or duodeno-duodenal bypass. A vagotomy and gastro-enterostomy should be avoided because they may compound the problem of diarrhoea.

Colonic disease

The management of colonic Crohn's disease remains controversial. A proportion of cases will have fulminating colitis, indistinguishable from ulcerative colitis. These cases should be managed with a colectomy, ileostomy and mucous fistula. Less severe cases may be improved by a split ileostomy, where diversion of the faecal stream may allow sufficient recovery of the colonic disease to allow later restoration of the continuity without resection. Localized segmental disease can be treated by conservative resection and anastomosis.

If there is diffuse colonic involvement but relative sparing of the rectum and no perianal disease, an ileorectal anastomosis will save the patient an ileostomy. There is some evidence, however, that these patients are more likely to develop a recurrence than those treated by an immediate proctocolectomy and ileostomy.

Perianal disease

In patients with perianal disease, as with gut involvement, it is important that surgery is kept to a minimum. Perianal fistulae and chronic fissures are often painless and even minor sphincter divisions in patients with a tendency to loose stools can result in troublesome incontinence. No treatment is necessary in about 40% of cases. Perianal abscesses must obviously be drained, but fistulae do not necessarily have to be laid open, and limited surgery is to be preferred. Only rarely will a proctectomy be necessary for severe perianal disease. Defunction by ileostomy may give temporary relief but in the long term it will not always arrest the disease. Strictures can be managed by gentle dilatation, and incontinence following fistula surgery may require sphincter repair.

Special problems

The elderly

In these patients, the distal colon and rectum are more commonly affected and there is an increased incidence of acute complications. Perianal disease can be troublesome but again it should be managed conservatively as far as possible.

Crohn's disease presenting as appendicitis

In patients thought to have appendicitis in whom terminal ileal Crohn's disease is found, the appendix should be removed. The ileal disease can be treated conservatively (medically) if it is not severe, but in advanced disease immediate resection is wise.

Abscess

Crohn's disease has become the most frequent cause of psoas abscess. This usually arises from a segment of terminal ileal disease densely adherent to the psoas sheet, with liquefaction of a portion of the underlying muscle. Following ileal resection, the abscess cavity must be debrided and drained using an indwelling catheter, which may have to be left in place for some time.

Fistulae to bladder or vagina

Fistulae to the bladder or vagina may arise from any part of the affected bowel (Fig. 8.6). Primary repair is not usually successful. Resection of the involved bowel is necessary together with repair of the fistula, and a covering ileostomy may be advisable. Some rectovaginal fistulae produce few symptoms and can be left untreated.

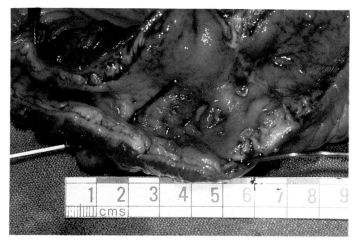

Fig. 8.6 Resected segment of ileal Crohn's disease which had fistulated into the bladder — the tract of the fistula is shown by the probe.

Cancer

Malignant change has now been reported in segments of chronic ileal disease, colonic disease and perianal fistulae. Surgeons managing patients with chronic disease should bear this in mind when dealing with long-standing strictures and fistulae.

FURTHER READING

de Silva H J, Kettlewell M S W, Mortensen N J, Jewell D P 1991 Acute inflammation in ileal pouches (pouchitis). Eur J Gastroenterol Hepatol 3: 343–349

Jewell D P, Caprilli R, Mortensen N, Nichols R J, Wright J P 1991 Indications and timing of surgery for severe ulcerative colitis. Gastroenterol Int 4: 141–164

Lee E C G (ed) 1987 Surgery of inflammatory bowel disease. Churchill Livingstone, Edinburgh.

9 Prognosis

ULCERATIVE COLITIS

Mortality

The mortality of ulcerative colitis is highest in the first year after diagnosis and in the first year after radical surgery. The principal causes of death are perforation and sepsis, uncontrolled haemorrhage, thromboembolism and malignancy. However, in a specialist centre, the mortality of a severe attack, including surgical mortality, should be less than 2%. Overall, the most recent studies have shown no difference between the mortality rate of patients with ulcerative colitis and a control population.

Morbidity

The complications of ulcerative colitis generally develop during the first two years of the disease, when mortality and the likelihood of colectomy are higher. Children and adolescents tend to run a more severe course. The major problems are colitis which fails to respond to adequate medical treatment, and severe colitis which still carries a high morbidity. Surgery for severe colitis is more hazardous than elective planned procedures.

Chronic anaemia from blood loss and colitis controlled only by high doses of oral steroids are sometimes indications for surgery, which will eventually be necessary in 15–20% of all patients who have ulcerative colitis.

However, it should be emphasized that most patients are able to maintain their normal occupation and enjoy a full social life.

Extent of disease

For patients with proctosigmoiditis followed over ten years, the disease remains localized to the rectum in 90%, with an excellent prognosis. Extension to the proximal colon occurs in about 10%. In patients with total colitis, there is a higher risk of surgery and serious complications.

Surgical problems

Operative mortality

For elective procedures, an operative mortality of 1% can be expected, but in emergency cases this may be as high as 10%.

Immediate postoperative period

1. *Perineal wound infection.* Complete healing can be expected in 60% of perineal wounds following a proctocolectomy. However, some patients develop troublesome perineal infection which may cause delayed healing.

2. *Ileostomy problems.* Necrosis and fistulae are rare complications, requiring refashioning of the stoma. Diarrhoea is common immediately after a stoma is fashioned but this usually resolves to around 500 ml stoma fluid per day. Skin problems around the stoma have become less common with the advent of better appliances and stoma therapy advisers.

3. *Intestinal obstruction.* Mechanical intestinal obstruction occurs in 10% of patients within a few years of operation. This is usually due to adhesions or bolus obstruction. Obstructive symptoms are managed by nasogastric suction, intravenous fluids and observation, but sometimes they require laparotomy.

Late morbidity

Disturbed sexual function

This may arise after a proctocolectomy in one of three ways. The most common sexual problem is psychogenic in origin. This may arise because the patient becomes embarrassed or fears that an ileostomy will make them less sexually attractive. Neurogenic disturbances due to injury to pelvic nerves during rectal dissection can occur, but they virtually never occur when care is taken with close dissection of the rectum during the colectomy. Perineal or vaginal scarring may make intercourse painful in a small minority of patients. Sexual dysfunction is more common in men than women, particularly in men over 50 years of age, which suggests that the major cause is psychogenic.

Perineal sinus

Delayed healing of a proctectomy wound may lead to a chronic perineal sinus in a minority of patients. This may require repeated curettage and occasionally grafting.

It should be stressed, however, that once a patient has had a successful proctocolectomy their life expectancy is very similar to that of the normal population.

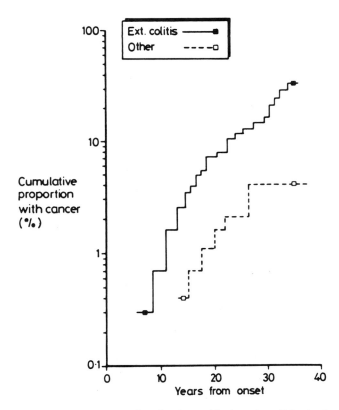

Fig. 9.1 The cumulative proportion of patients with ulcerative colitis who develop a colonic cancer during the course of the disease. The risk is seen predominantly in those with extensive colitis (solid line). Reproduced from Gyde et al., Gut 29: 206–217; 1988

Cancer risk

The risk of colorectal cancer occurs in patients with extensive colitis who have had the disease for more than ten years and who have pursued a chronic, continuous course. The risk is about 7% at 20 years, and 16% at 30 years (Fig. 9.1). There is little or no increased risk for those with distal disease. The prognosis of cancer complicating colitis is probably similar to that in patients without colitis.

Surveillance programmes have been developed for patients with long-standing total colitis. An annual or biennial colonoscopy is performed from ten years after diagnosis. At colonoscopy, the colonic mucosa is inspected for the presence of suspicious or raised lesions (Fig. 9.2) and these are biopsied together with random

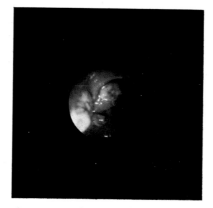

Fig. 9.2 Irregular polyps seen at colonoscopy in a patient with a total ulcerative colitis for 17 years. Biopsy specimens showed high-grade dysplasia as well as frank malignant change.

samples taken throughout the length of the colon. These biopsies are examined for the pre-malignant changes of dysplasia (Fig. 9.3), and where these changes are severe (high-grade) a proctocolectomy may have to be recommended. Although the considerable expense and logistic problems of colitis surveillance have been questioned, most major centres offer such programmes to their patients with ulcerative colitis.

CROHN'S DISEASE

Recurrent disease

The presence or absence of macroscopic change at the margins of a resection do not affect recurrence rates after surgery for Crohn's

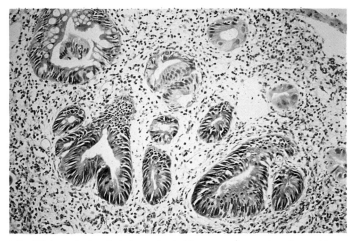

Fig. 9.3   High-grade dysplasia in a colonic biopsy specimen taken from a 34-year-old man who had had a total colitis from the age of 16. There is glandular distortion, stratification of the epithelium and marked pleiomorphism and hyperchromaticism of the nuclei.

disease, neither does the presence nor the absence of microscopic granulomata. The clinical recurrence rate is 50% at ten years and 25% will require a second operation. The recurrence rate is lower after proctocolectomy. However, colonoscopic and histological evidence suggests that at least 75% of patients will develop new lesions in the neoterminal ileum within 1 year of resection. If these new lesions are severe, they predict a high rate of clinical recurrence.

Cancer risk

Anecdotal examples of carcinoma of the small and large bowel and anus have been reported and there is growing evidence for an increased cancer risk in Crohn's disease, but the degree of risk has not yet been determined. Dysplasia occurs in Crohn's colitis but its incidence has not yet been defined. It remains unclear whether patients with long-standing colonic Crohn's disease should be offered surveillance similar to that given to patients with ulcerative colitis.

Overall prognosis

About a quarter of all cases are diagnosed before the age of 21 years. The cumulative risk of death is increased two-fold during long-term follow-up. A study in Birmingham suggested a cumulative relative risk of ten times in the first five years after diagnosis, falling to 2.4-fold at 15 years. However, this was not true in Oxford, where the excess mortality was only seen after 15 years of having the disease. Although the mortality is low, there is a significant morbidity. Thus, about 70% of patients will require at least one operation during their lifetime, with an average of about 1.5 bowel resections per patient. Nevertheless, the quality of life for the vast majority of patients is good in between episodes of active disease and many remain well for years before the disease relapses or a complication, such as a stricture, develops.

FURTHER READING

Farmer R G, Whelan G, Fazio V W 1985 Long-term follow-up of patients with Crohn's disease: relationship between the clinical pattern and prognosis. Gastroenterology 88: 1818–1825

Hendriksen C, Kreiner S, Binder V 1985 Long-term prognosis in ulcerative colitis — based on results from a regional patient group from the County of Copenhagen. Gut 26: 158–163

Lennard-Jones J E, Melville D M, Morson B D, Ritchie J K, Williams C B 1990 Pre-cancer and cancer in extensive ulcerative colitis: findings among 401 patients over 22 years. Gut 31: 800–806

Prior P, Gyde S, Cooke W T, Waterhouse J A H, Allan R N 1981 Mortality in Crohn's disease. Gastroenterology 80: 307–312

Riddell R H, Goldman H, Ransohoff D F et al 1983 Standardized nomenclature, terminology and criteria for dysplasia in inflammatory bowel disease with recommendations for patient management. Hum Pathol 14: 931–968

Truelove S C, Pena A S 1976 Course and prognosis of Crohn's disease. Gut 17: 196–201

Useful addresses

National Association for Colitis and Crohn's Disease
98A London Road
St Albans
Herts
AL1 1NX

Crohn's in Childhood Research Association (CIRCA)
56A Uxbridge Road
Shepherd's Bush
London
W12 8LP

Ileostomy Association of Great Britain and Ireland
Amblehurst House
Chobham
Woking
Surrey
GU24 8PZ

British Colostomy Association
15 Station Road
Reading
Berks
RG1 1LG

The British Digestive Foundation
Room D
7 Chandos Street
Cavendish Square
London
W1A 2LN

Index

Aetiology/pathogenesis
  dietary factors, 10
  environmental factors, 9–13
  genetic factors, 9
  infective agents, 9–10
Age/sex, and incidence, 7
Albumin, serum levels, 23, 32
5-Aminosalicylic acid (5-ASA), 52–53, 63
  enema, 50
Amoebiasis, 21
Amoebic colitis, 31
Amyloidosis, 48
Anaemia
  Crohn's disease, 18, 32
  hypochromic microcytic, 21
  ulcerative colitis, 15
Anal tags, 19
Ankylosing spondylitis, HLA-B27 association, 44
Anterior uveitis, 45
Antidiarrhoeal agents, 55, 63
Antigen-antibody reactions, 11
Aphthous ulcers
  chronic, 33, 37, 38
  oral, 18
  rectal, 33
Appendicitis, and Crohn's disease, 67
Arthropathy, 43–45
Associations and societies, addresses, 75
Augmentin, 63
Azathioprine, 52, 55

Barium enemas
  Crohn's disease, 33–34, 35, 36, 37, 38
  double-contrast, and perforation, 25
  ulcerative colitis, 25–30
Behçet's disease, 40
Bile salt, malabsorption, 54
Bladder fistulae, Crohn's disease, 68

C-reactive protein, 23, 32
Calcium oxalate kidney stones, 48
Campylobacter jejuni, 21
Cancer
  and Crohn's disease, 68
  risks
    Crohn's disease, 73
    ulcerative colitis, 71, 72
  see also Cholangiocarcinoma; Dysplasias
Candidiasis, oral, 15
Children, treatment, 56
Cholangiocarcinoma, 46, 48
Cholangitis, primary sclerosing, 23, 46–48
Cholesterol gallstones, 46
Cholestyramine, 55
Clinical features
  Crohn's disease, 17–20
  ulcerative colitis, 14–17
Clostridium difficile, 21
Codeine phosphate, 55, 63
Colectomy, severe ulcerative colitis, 51
Colitis
  fulminant, 66
    stool appearances, 14–15
  granulomatous, 4
Colon
  acute dilatation, ulcerative colitis, 17
  haustral pattern, 25, 26–27, 29
  inflammatory infiltrate, ulcerative colitis, 1–2
  perforation, ulcerative colitis, 17
Colonic Crohn's disease, 4
  surgery, 66
Colonoscopy
  Crohn's disease, 36–37, 39, 40
  ulcerative colitis, 28
Complement activation, 11

Complications
    Crohn's disease, surgery, 64
    ulcerative colitis, 16–17
    postoperative, 70
Conjunctivitis, 45
Corticosteroids
    acute ulcerative colitis, 49, 50
    Crohn's disease, 54–55
    mortality reduction, 4–5
Crohn's disease, 31
    as appendicitis, 67
    definition, 2–4
    postsurgical recurrence, 54
    sites/clinical picture, 17–18
    terminology, 4
Crypt abscesses, 2
Cyclosporin, Crohn's disease, 55
Cytokines, release effects, 13
Cytomegalovirus infection, 32

Diarrhoea, nocturnal, 14
Diet
    aetiological aspects, 10
    Crohn's disease therapy, 55–56
    and disease progression/relapse, 56
    elemental, 10, 56
Differential diagnosis
    Crohn's disease, 40
    ulcerative colitis, 30–32
Drug treatment, Crohn's disease, 54–55
Duodenal Crohn's disease, surgery, 66
Dysplasias
    Crohn's colitis, 73
    ulcerative colitis, 72, 73

Elderly, Crohn's disease, 67
Elemental diets, Crohn's disease, 10, 56
Elimination diets, food intolerance, 56
Enterocutaneous fistulae, Crohn's
    disease, 55, 56
Environmental factors
    aetiology/pathogenesis, 9–13
    incidence/prevalence, 7–8
Episcleritis, 45
Epithelial cells
    antigen presentation, 12
    function impairment, ulcerative
        colitis, 11
Erythema nodosum, 42
Erythrocyte sedimentation rate (ESR),
    23, 32
Ethnic associations, incidence/
    prevalence, 7, 8
Extraintestinal manifestations, 42–48
Eyes, disorders, 45

Failure to thrive, 18
Fatty liver, 45, 46
Finger clubbing, 15, 18
Food intolerance, elimination diets, 56

Gallstones, Crohn's disease, 46
Genetic factors, 9
Granulomas
    Crohn's disease, 3–4
    epithelioid, rectal, 38
Granulomatous colitis, 4
Growth stunting, 18

Hemicolectomy, limited right, ileal
    Crohn's disease, 65
Hepatitis, chronic active, 46
Hepatobiliary manifestations, 45–48
Herpes simplex, 32
Historical aspects, 4–5
HIV infection, colonic disorders, 32
HLA-B27 association, ankylosing
    spondylitis, 44
HLA-DR association, ulcerative colitis,
    9, 12
Hydrocortisone
    Crohn's disease, 54
    ulcerative colitis, 50, 51
Hyperoxaluria, 48
Hypoproteinaemia, 15, 18

IgG, 11
IgM, 11
Ileal Crohn's disease, surgery, 65–66
Ileitis, acute, 19–20
Ileorectal anastomosis, ulcerative colitis,
    59–60
Ileostomy
    Kock pouch, 59
    problems, 70
    and proctocolectomy, ulcerative
        colitis, 58
Immune pathways, activation, 12–13
Immunological findings, 11–13
Immunoregulatory control, disturbance,
    12
Incidence/prevalence
    age/sex, 7
    Crohn's disease, 6–7
    environmental factors, 7–8
    ethnic associations, 7, 8
    familial, 9
    geographical variations, 6–7, 8
    social class, 7, 11
    ulcerative colitis, 6

Indium-111 autologous neutrophil
   scanning, 34–36, 39
   advantages/disadvantages, 35–36
Infective agents, aetiology/pathogenesis,
   9–10
Infective colitis, 31
Infertility, sulphasalazine-related, 53
Inflammatory bowel disease, 1
Inflammatory infiltrate, colonic, 1–2
Intestinal obstruction, postoperative, 70
Investigations
   Crohn's disease, 32–40
   ulcerative colitis, 21–32
Iron deficiency
   Crohn's disease, 18, 32, 54
   ulcerative colitis, 15
Irritable bowel syndrome, 19–20
Ischaemic colitis, 31

Johne's disease, 10
Joints, disorders, 43–45

Kaposi's sarcoma, 32
Kock continent ileostomy, ulcerative
   colitis, 59

Laboratory investigations
   Crohn's disease, 32
   ulcerative colitis, 21–23
Liver function tests, ulcerative colitis, 23
Loperamide, 55, 63

Macrophages, inflammatory mediator
   release effects, 13
Malabsorption, Crohn's disease, 18
Medical management
   Crohn's disease, 53–57
   ulcerative colitis, 49–53
6-Mercaptopurine, 55
Mesalazine, 50, 52–53
Metronidazole, 55, 63
Milk-free diets, ulcerative colitis, 10
Morbidity, ulcerative colitis, 69
   late, 70–72
Mortality
   and corticosteroids, 4–5
   postoperative, 70
   ulcerative colitis, 69, 70
Mycobacterium avium intracellulare, 32
Mycobacterium paratuberculosis, Crohn's
   disease, 9–10

Nephrolithiasis, 48
Neutrophils, autologous, Indium-111
   labelled, scanning, 34–36, 39

Olsalazine, 53
Oral contraceptive pill, and disease
   incidence, 10–11
Orosomucoid concentrations, serum, 23,
   32
Osteomalacia, 18

Pelvic pouch
   pouchitis, 62–63
   types, 60–61
   ulcerative colitis, 60–63
Perianal Crohn's disease, surgery, 67
Perianal fistula, 19, 20
Pericholangitis, 46
Perineal sinus, postoperative, 71
Perineal wound infection,
   proctocolectomy, 70
Physical signs
   Crohn's disease, 18–19
   ulcerative colitis, 15
Plasma cells, IgG and IgM, 11
Postoperative complications, ulcerative
   colitis, 70
Pouchitis, 62–63
Prednisolone
   Crohn's disease, 54
   and elemental diets, 56
   ulcerative colitis, 50, 51
Pregnancy, and inflammatory bowel
   disease, 57
Primary sclerosing cholangitis, 23, 46–48
   aetiology, 47–48
   diagnosis, 47
Proctitis
   chlamydial, 32
   gonococcal, 32
   haemorrhage, 14
   medical management, 49–50
Proctocolectomy
   and ileostomy, ulcerative colitis, 58
   restorative, pouch operation, 60–63
   ulcerative colitis, 58, 60–63
Proctosigmoiditis, prognosis, 69–70
Prognosis
   Crohn's disease, 72–74
   ulcerative colitis, 69–72
   and disease extent, 69–70
Pseudomembraneous colitis, 31
Pseudopolyps, ulcerative colitis, 27–30
Psoas abscesses, Crohn's disease, 67
Pyoderma gangrenosum, 42–43

Quality of life, Crohn's disease, 74

Radiology
  Crohn's disease, 33–34, 35, 36, 37, 38
  ulcerative colitis, 23–27, 28, 29
Rectal biopsy
  Crohn's disease, 38–39
  ulcerative colitis, 28–29
Recurrent Crohn's disease, 54, 72–73
Regional enteritis, 4
Regional ileitis, 4

Sacroiliitis, 44
Septicaemia, ulcerative colitis, 16
Severity assessment, ulcerative colitis, 16
Sexual function, disorders,
    postoperative, 70–71
Short bowel syndrome, 55, 64, 65
Sigmoidoscopy
  Crohn's disease, 32–33
  ulcerative colitis, 23–24
Skin disorders, 42–43
Skip lesions, Crohn's disease, 3
Small bowel
  adhesions, 63
  cobblestone appearance, 33, 34, 35
Smoking, and disease incidence, 10, 11
Social class, and incidence, 7, 11
Sphincter-saving operations, 60–63
Steatorrhoea, 18
Stool examination
  Crohn's disease, 32
  ulcerative colitis, 21
Strictureplasty, ileal Crohn's disease,
    65–66
Sulphasalazine
  Crohn's disease, 54
  proctitis, 49, 50
  remission maintenance, 52–53
  side-effects, 52, 53

Surgery
  Crohn's disease, 64–68
    indications, 64
  emergency, ulcerative colitis, 63
  ulcerative colitis, 58–63
Surgical problems, ulcerative colitis, 70
Symptoms
  Crohn's disease, 17–18
  ulcerative colitis, 14–15

Tachycardia, 15, 19
T-helper cells, B-cell uncontrolled
    interaction, 12
Thrombocytosis, 23
Thromboembolism, 16, 48
Total parenteral nutrition, 55
Toxic dilatation, acute, 25
T-suppressor cells, intra-epithelial, 12
Tuberculosis, ileocaecal, 40

Ulcerative colitis
  acute, medical therapy, 49, 50
  definition, 1–2, 4
  mild attacks, 50
  moderate attacks, 51
  refractory, 52
  severe attacks, 51
Uveitis, anterior, 45

Vaginal fistulae, Crohn's disease, 68
Vitamin B_{12} deficiency, 32, 54

Water/electrolyte deficiencies, ulcerative
    colitis, 16
Wound infection, proctocolectomy, 70

Yersinia infections, terminal ileitis, 40